Statistics for Pharmacists

Alain Li Wan Po
BPharm, BA, PhD, FPSNI, FRSC, FRPharmS, FRSS

Professor of Clinical Pharmaceutics
The University of Nottingham

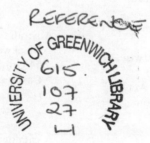

**Blackwell
Science**

© 1998 by
Blackwell Science Ltd
Editorial Offices:
Osney Mead, Oxford OX2 0EL
25 John Street, London WC1N 2BL
23 Ainslie Place, Edinburgh EH3 6AJ
350 Main Street, Malden
  MA 02148 5018, USA
54 University Street, Carlton
  Victoria 3053, Australia

Other Editorial Offices:

Blackwell Wissenschafts-Verlag GmbH
Kurfürstendamm 57
10707 Berlin, Germany

Blackwell Science KK
MG Kodenmacho Building
7–10 Kodenmacho Nihombashi
Chuo-ku, Tokyo 104, Japan

First published 1997

Set in 10 on 12 pt Times
by Best-set Typesetter Ltd, Hong Kong
Printed and bound in Great Britain by
MPG Books Limited, Bodmin, Cornwall

The Blackwell Science logo is a
trade mark of Blackwell Science Ltd,
registered at the United Kingdom
Trade Marks Registry

DISTRIBUTORS

Marston Book Services Ltd
PO Box 269
Abingdon
Oxon OX14 4YN
(*Orders*:   Tel: 01235 465500
             Fax: 01235 465555)

USA
Blackwell Science, Inc.
Commerce Place
350 Main Street
Malden, MA 02148 5018
(*Orders*:   Tel: 800 759 6102
                    617 388 8250
             Fax: 617 388 8255)

Canada
Copp Clark Professional
200 Adelaide Street West, 3rd Floor
Toronto, Ontario M5H 1W7
(*Orders*:   Tel: 416 597-1616
                    800 815 9417
             Fax: 416 597 1617)

Australia
Blackwell Science Pty Ltd
54 University Street
Carlton, Victoria 3053
(*Orders*:   Tel: 03 9347 0300
             Fax: 03 9347 5001)

A catalogue record for this title
is available from the British Library

ISBN 0-632–04881-6

Library of Congress
Cataloging-in-Publication Data
is available

Contents

Preface

Most pharmacy students are taught some statistics during their undergraduate studies. Yet very few progress to become proficient at using statistics for evaluating their data. I believe that this is due to several factors:

1 statistical concepts are often difficult;
2 the amount of time given to the teaching of statistics in the average pharmacy degree is usually too short;
3 statistics textbooks aimed at pharmacy students are often too limited in scope or alternatively are too mathematically detailed;
4 textbooks often box statistical methods too rigidly by, for example, restricting discussion to parametric or non-parametric tests and
5 the teaching of statistics is often too compartmentalised and is therefore often seen as an unnecessary add-on by pharmacy students.

I hope that this book will help the student overcome some of these difficulties and will serve as a bridge between introductory texts which do not go much beyond the Student's *t*-test and the mathematically detailed treatises which pharmacy under-graduates generally find too demanding. I have attempted to adopt a more holistic approach to the use of statistics than is the case in many introductory texts. In particular, I have discussed parametric and non-parametric tests side-by-side. In my experience the major difficulty that students find in the use of statistics is how to choose an appropriate test for their proposed studies and what pitfalls they should watch out for. I have, therefore, provided (where appropriate) a test selection flow diagram which I hope readers will find useful.

In line with the increased emphasis on estimation, an extensive discussion of confidence interval and sample size is given. Survival analysis is also introduced because of its growing importance in the pharmaceutical sciences.

I have detailed the algebraic manipulations associated with the use of particular statistical methods to give the reader an appreciation of the underlying principles. It is not my intention that the reader should reproduce those calculations but rather that they would be in a position to better interpret computer outputs.

The use of computer packages is illustrated with two of the most popular and versatile statistical software packages currently available, MINITAB (a registered trade mark of MINITAB Inc.) and SAS (a registered trade mark of the SAS Institute). The former is a particularly user-friendly package while the latter is an industry-standard in many fields because of its comprehensiveness.

I would greatly appreciate comments about any aspect of the book.

Chapter 1
Perspectives, Definitions and Data Description

1.1 What is statistics?

Statistics is a branch of mathematics dealing with the presentation and analysis of numerical data. The two main branches of statistics are *descriptive statistics* and *inferential statistics*. Descriptive statistics attempt to present data in numerical, graphical or tabular form in order to convey information clearly. With inferential statistics attempts are made to draw conclusions from results of investigational studies. Usually inferences are made about populations from sample data.

1.2 What are statistical populations and samples?

In statistics a *population* is the set of all experimental units or measurements of interest to the investigator in a particular study. For example, in studying the incidence of caries among 10-year-old children in England, the population would be all 10-year-old children in England. If the study involves comparing the incidence of caries among 10-year-olds in England and Scotland then a second population, made up of all 10-year-olds in Scotland, would be required. As a further example, in studying tablet defects in one production run, the population would be all tablets produced in that run. Figure 1.1 illustrates the concept of a statistical population further. Clearly it is not possible to examine every 10-year-old in a population as large as in England, nor is it feasible to inspect every tablet in a production run. To make the work manageable, *samples* are studied.

1.3 What types of data can statistics be applied to?

The statistical analysis appropriate for a set of data will depend on the type of data being considered and generally four types can be identified:

- *Nominal or categorical data*: With such data classification can only be into groups. No ranking is possible. Examples include classification according to sex, religious affiliation, disease severity, cancer type or racial groupings. The

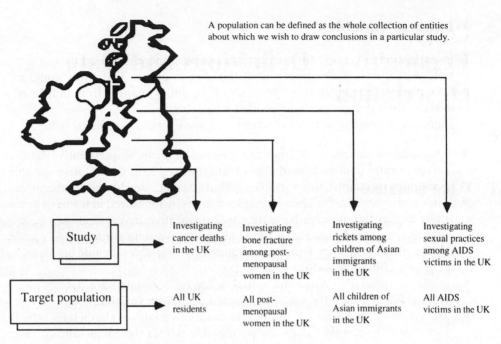

A population can be defined as the whole collection of entities about which we wish to draw conclusions in a particular study.

| Study | Investigating cancer deaths in the UK | Investigating bone fracture among post-menopausal women in the UK | Investigating rickets among children of Asian immigrants in the UK | Investigating sexual practices among AIDS victims in the UK |

| Target population | All UK residents | All post-menopausal women in the UK | All children of Asian immigrants in the UK | All AIDS victims in the UK |

Fig. 1.1 Nature of a 'statistical' population.

categories are often restricted to two (e.g. male/female; alive/dead; symptom present or absent). Such data are said to be *binary*.

- *Ordinal data*:   Rank ordering of the data is possible. Examples include classification into groupings such as worse, no change and better or small, medium and large or absent, mild and severe. In each case classification into any of the alternatives will carry a clear quantitative significance in that absent is clearly understood to be less bad than mild which in turn is less bad than severe, if the classification refers to an unpleasant symptom.

- *Interval data*:   Such data, in addition to being suitable for classification into rank order can also be precisely defined in measured units relative to each other. Examples include temperature data.

- *Ratio data*:   Such data are of an even higher order than interval data since, in addition to being well defined, in measured units, relative to each other, ratios of the data also convey precise quantitative information. Thus the ratio 100°C:50°C does not mean that 100°C is twice as hot as 50°C. Temperatures are therefore interval data not ratio data. Height, weight and length are ratio data since 2 metres is clearly understood to be twice as long as 1 metre and 2 kilograms is clearly twice 1 kilogram in weight. An important point to note also is that ratio data have a true zero point. Thus 0 height means absence of height. On the other hand 0°C does not mean no temperature. In the present discussion interval data and ratio data will be used interchangeably.

1.4   What is a 'variable'?

In investigating any entity for quantitative analysis, there is a need to measure or to note a property or characteristic of the chosen entity. The entity could be a person, place or an object. If the property of the entity changes from individual to individual, then that property is labelled a *variable*.

There are a number of types of variable, some of which are listed below:

- *Quantitative variables*:   Variables measured in terms of quantitative data (interval or ratio data as defined above), are referred to as quantitative variables. Examples of quantitative variables include height, weight and temperature.
- *Qualitative variables*:   These variables cannot be measured in terms of precise units as can the quantitative data. Only qualitative descriptions can be used and the measurements are in terms of qualitative data (ordinal and nominal data as defined above). Examples of qualitative variables include ethnic group, religious affiliation and sex.
- *Random variable*:   When the values taken by a variable are determined by chance factors, then the variable is called a random variable.
- *Discrete random variable*:   A discrete random variable is characterised by the fact that only certain values are permissible within the range studied. Thus, if one were studying the number of teeth at specific ages, the number of teeth can only take whole numbers. Fractional numbers would not make sense. Likewise if one were measuring number of deaths, fractional deaths are clearly ridiculous.
- *Continuous random variable*:   In this case, the number of possible values is infinite within the range studied. Thus, height or blood pressure is a continuous variable in that, no matter how close the blood pressures or heights of two individuals are, it is theoretically possible to find one individual with intermediate values.

1.5   What is a 'statistical' sample?

A sample is a part of the population under study. In statistics one is usually interested in a sample which is representative of the population concerned. For example, if one were to study the incidence of bone fractures among post-menopausal women, a sample of such women selected from, say, a small town where most women work at sedentary jobs would not be representative of the whole population of post-menopausal women since physical activity is known to affect bone density. Likewise in a study of rickets, a sample of children of Asian immigrants drawn from a town in which most Asians come from Pakistan would not be representative of the Asian immigrant population as a whole, since there are wide differences even among different Asian groups. Infant mortality, for example, is known to be higher among Bangladeshi immigrants than among Pakistani immigrants.

1.6   How can a representative sample be drawn?

Ensuring that a sample is representative of a population under study is often quite difficult, but a number of well-defined techniques are available to ensure this as far as possible and these will be exemplified with survey sampling.

- *Simple random sampling*:   In such a scheme, one attempts to ensure that each individual in the target population has an equal chance of being sampled and the selection of any member of the population concerned does not affect the chance of any of the other remaining members of the population from being selected.

    Ensuring randomness is an essential feature of such random sampling. Randomness is usually achieved by using a *sampling frame* composed of a list of all the members of the target population and then choosing a sample at random with the help of a table of random numbers or a random number generator. The electoral register, for example, is often used as a sampling frame for many studies although it becomes rapidly out of date. Great care is required in choosing a sample. Thus, in investigating whether medical advice could be satisfactorily given via the telephone, a telephone directory may be an acceptable sample frame but the same directory would be unsuitable for investigating personality traits since individuals who are ex-directory and those without telephones would be left out.

- *Systematic random sample*:   Simple random sampling is time-consuming and expensive. An alternative quicker and cheaper method is systematic random sampling. In essence one chooses a *random start* and then all the subsequent choices are made at a fixed *sampling interval*. For example, one may decide to choose 1 in 10 from a given population. The first choice could be item 07 from the first 10 items. Subsequently the choices would be items 17, 27, 37, 47 . . . Note, however, that with this type of sampling, if the list making up the sampling frame is structured, then very unrepresentative samples will be produced.

- *Stratified sample*:   Stratified sampling is usually performed in order to reduce sampling error. The population is categorised into *strata* and samples are taken from each stratum in proportion to its true representation in the population. For example, in investigating hip fractures in post-menopausal women stratification into age groups may improve the estimates made. Note that the strata are mutually exclusive.

- *Cluster sampling*:   This type of sampling is actually used to reduce costs. This is achieved by restricting the sample to a limited number of geographical areas (clusters) which are thought to be representative of the whole population. For example, in investigating infant mortality, clusters may be chosen using areas which, among Asian immigrant children, are known to have a good mix of the different Asian immigrant subgroups. Sampling error is usually larger with cluster sampling than with stratified sampling.

1.7   How should a sample or a population be described?

Most investigators would be interested in knowing about the value to which the sample or population would centre round. In statistics three common measures of this central tendency are used:

(1)   The arithmetic *mean* – the sum of all observations divided by the number of observations

$$\bar{x} = \sum x_i / n.$$ (1.1)

(2)   The *median* – this is the value or observation which subdivides the numerically ordered data into two equal halves. If the number of observations is an odd number, then the median is the middle observation. The median of an even number of observations is given by the mean of the two middle values. The median is a more useful measure of central tendency than the mean when the underlying population is non-symmetrical.

(3)   The *mode* – the observation which occurs most frequently in the set of data studied. It is obvious that the mode may sometimes not be single-valued. The mode is not often used but an interesting application is in the study of polymorphic drug metabolism when the mode can be shown to undergo marked shifts in certain cases.

A better feel for a data set will be gained if, in addition to an indication of its central tendency, a measure of its spread is also given. For any single value, x_i, its deviation from the mean is given by $(x_i - \bar{x})$. To present each of these deviations would be confusing to the reader. Their sum equals zero and is therefore not useful. A more useful measure is the sum of their squared deviations

$$\sum \left(x_i - \bar{x}\right)^2$$

since each squared deviation will be a positive value. One problem, however, remains since the sum of squared deviations will depend on the number of observations. If the spreads of two samples are to be compared, then there is a need to standardise. With samples it is usual to standardise by $(n - 1)$ where n is the number of observations. This standardised measure of spread of a population is called the *variance*, s^2.

$$s^2 = \sum \left(x_i - \bar{x}\right)^2 / \left(n - 1\right)$$ (1.2)

The *standard deviation* is the positive square root of the variance. By taking the square root, the units are returned back to those of the original measurements.

The *standard error* is the standard deviation of an estimate. Thus, the standard error of the mean (SEM) is the standard deviation of the mean. If s is the standard deviation of a sample then the SEM is given by the formula

$$\text{SEM} = s/\sqrt{n} \tag{1.3}$$

1.8   What is the coefficient of variation?

The ratio of the standard deviation to the mean is the *coefficient of variation* (CV). This statistic is usually expressed as a percentage. Therefore $\text{CV} = 100(s/\bar{x})$. A coefficient of variation of 5% means that the standard deviation is equal to 5% of the mean ($\bar{x}$).

1.9   What are other measures used to define the spread of data?

To define the spread of data around the average value, other measures used include *quartiles*, *deciles* and *percentiles*. These measures are the appropriate ones to use when the population is non-symmetrical.

The *quartiles* subdivide the data set in such a way that 25% of the values are above the *upper quartile* (Q_U) and 25% are below the *lower quartile* (Q_L). For the *deciles*, 10% of the values are above the upper decile and 10% below the lower decile. The upper quartile is the 75th *percentile* and the upper decile is the 90th percentile. The *interquartile range* dQ is given by $Q_U - Q_L$. The *mid-interquartile* range is given by $(Q_U - Q_L)$. The *range* is given by the interval between the two extreme values E_L and E_U.

The lower and upper quartile values can be calculated according to the following definitions:

(1)   When n, the number of points in the data set, is divisible by 4. The lower quartile is given by the arithmetic mean of the $(n/4)^{\text{th}}$ and the $(n/4 + 1)^{\text{th}}$ values. Similarly, the upper quartile is given by the arithmetic mean of the $(3n/4)^{\text{th}}$ and the $(3n/4 + 1)^{\text{th}}$ value.

(2)   When n, the number of points in the data set, is not divisible by 4. The lower quartile is given by the value corresponding to the next integer from $(n/4)$. Similarly, the upper quartile is given by the value corresponding to the next whole integer from $(3n/4)$.

Example 1.1
For data set 1, where n is divisible by 4, calculate the lower and upper quartiles.

Solution
Data set 1: X: x_1, x_2, x_3, x_4, x_5, x_6, x_7, x_8, x_9, x_{10}, x_{11}, x_{12}

$$\text{Lower quartile} = \frac{x_3 + x_4}{2} \qquad \text{Upper quartile} = \frac{x_9 + x_{10}}{2}$$

Example 1.2
For data set 2, where n is *not* divisible by 4, calculate the lower and upper quartiles.

Solution

Data set 2: X: x_1, x_2, x_3, x_4, x_5, x_6, x_7, x_8, x_9, x_{10}, x_{11}

Lower quartile = x_3 Upper quartile = x_9

Example 1.3

Example 1.3 gives some derived statistics for data set 3.

Data set 3: X: 25, 26, 26, 30, 32, 36, 38, 38, 38, 39, 40, 52
$n = 12$

$$\text{Median} = \frac{(n/2)^{\text{th}} + (n/2 + 1)^{\text{th}} \text{ values}}{2} = \frac{36 + 38}{2} = 37$$

$$\text{Upper quartile} = \frac{(3n/4)^{\text{th}} + (3n/4 + 1)^{\text{th}} \text{ values}}{2} = \frac{38 + 39}{2} = 38.5$$

$$\text{Lower quartile} = \frac{(n/4)^{\text{th}} + (n/4 + 1)^{\text{th}} \text{ values}}{2} = \frac{26 + 30}{2} = 28$$

Lower extreme $= E_L = 25$
Upper extreme $= E_U = 52$
Interquartile range $= Q_U - Q_L = 38.5 - 28 = 10.5$
Range $= E_U - E_L = 52 - 25 = 27$

Stem plot 1: The stem plot of data set 3 should be self-explanatory

2	5 6 6
3	0 2 6 8 8 8 9
4	0
5	2

where   2 | 5 represents 25. Thus, on the first level we have values 25, 26 and 26 from data set 3. The stem plot gives the reader a quick description of the distribution of the data.

The same stem plot would also represent data set 4:

Data set 4: X: 250, 260, 260, 300, 320, 360, 380, 380, 380, 390, 400, 520

The stem plot would be the same as stem plot 1. The footnote would, however, read 2|5 represents 250.

1.10   Graphical representation: single data set

The box plot is a useful graph for summarising data sets. Figure 1.2 shows the general features of a box plot. A box represents the data between the lower and

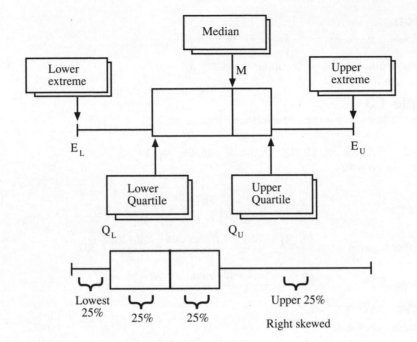

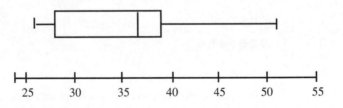

Fig. 1.2 Features of a box plot.

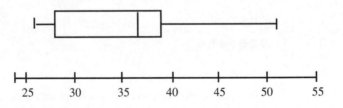

Fig. 1.3 Box plot of data set 3.

upper quartiles and lines (whiskers) are drawn to represent the lower and upper extremes. The median is represented by a line drawn across the box. Figure 1.3 shows a box plot drawn for data set 3 given in Example 1.3.

1.11   Graphs with MINITAB

To illustrate different types of plots that can be produced with MINITAB, a set of blood cholesterol measurements shown below is used as sample data.

```
MTB>SORT C1
MTB>PRINT C1

    Cholest
     2.9  3.2  3.5  3.6  3.6  3.7  3.8  3.8  3.8  3.9  3.9
     4.0  4.0  4.1  4.2  4.2  4.2  4.3  4.3  4.3  4.3  4.3
     4.4  4.4  4.4  4.4  4.4  4.4  4.4  4.4  4.4  4.5  4.5
     4.5  4.5  4.5  4.6  4.6  4.6  4.7  4.7  4.7  4.8  4.8
     4.9  4.9  4.9  5.0  5.0  5.1  5.1  5.2  5.2  5.2  5.2
     5.3  5.3  5.3  5.3  5.4  5.5  5.5  5.6  5.6  5.6  5.6
     5.7  5.7  5.8  5.8  5.8  6.0  6.2  6.2  6.2  6.3  6.3
     6.3  6.4  6.4  6.5  6.5  6.6  6.6  6.6  6.6  6.7  7.0
     7.0  7.2  7.4  7.5  7.5  7.6  7.8  7.9  7.9  7.9  8.0
     8.3  9.2  9.6
```

The SORT command sorts the data in increasing order. The PRINT command produces the set of cholesterol measurements previously entered into column 1 of a MINITAB worksheet.

1.11.1   Histogram

```
MTB>HISTOGRAM C1
Histogram of Cholest N = 102


    Midpoint Count
         3.0      2   **
         3.5      4   ****
         4.0     11   **********
         4.5     25   *************************
         5.0     13   *************
         5.5     13   *************
         6.0      7   *******
         6.5     12   ************
         7.0      3   ***
         7.5      4   ****
         8.0      5   *****
         8.5      1   *
         9.0      1   *
         9.5      1   *
```

Most readers will be familiar with the histogram. The standard plot gives the number of points under each column. The histogram gives a useful representation of the distribution of the observed values. The stem-and-leaf plot is, however, more informative (see section 1.11.2).

```
MTB>Ghistogram C1
```

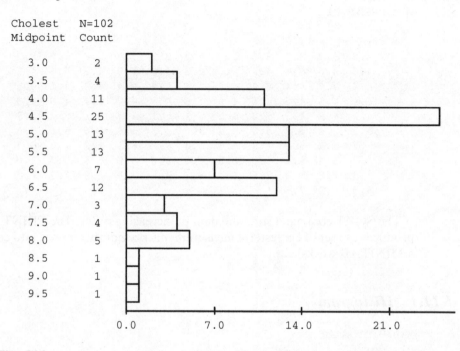

```
    Cholest    N=102
    Midpoint   Count

      3.0        2
      3.5        4
      4.0       11
      4.5       25
      5.0       13
      5.5       13
      6.0        7
      6.5       12
      7.0        3
      7.5        4
      8.0        5
      8.5        1
      9.0        1
      9.5        1

          0.0      7.0      14.0      21.0
```

The Ghistogram command produces the classical histogram as shown above.

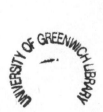

1.11.2   Stem-and-leaf plot

```
MTB>Stem and leaf C1

Stem-and-leaf of Cholest N = 102
Leaf Unit = 0.10

              Leaf Unit = 0.10
          1    2    9
          2    3    2
         11    3    566788899
         31    4    0012223333344444444
         47    4    5555566677788999
        (13)   5    0011222233334
         42    5    55666677888
         31    6    022233344
         22    6    5566667
         15    7    0024
         11    7    5568999
          4    8    03
          2    8
          2    9    2
          1    9    6
```

Cumulative number
of readings ──────────┘

└── Leaf (in the example the value
        given is the decimal unit)

└── Stem (in the example the value given
    is units)

The stem-and-leaf plot is essentially the same as a histogram except that the values included under each column are listed. Thus, the first column consists of one reading 2.9. The second column also has one reading only, 3.2. The third column has (11 – 2) or nine readings – (3.5, 3.6, 3.6, 3.7, 3.8, 3.8, 3.8, 3.9, 3.9) and so on. The stem-and-leaf plot is therefore much more informative than the histogram.

1.11.3   Dot plot

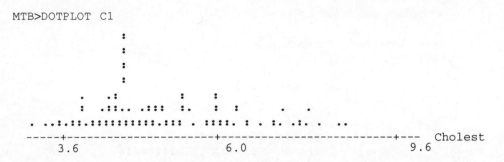

```
MTB>DOTPLOT C1
```

The dotplot provides similar information to the histogram but the axis is divided into more divisions and each data point is represented by a dot. Identical values are stacked.

1.11.4   Box plot

```
MTB> GBOXPLOT C1
```

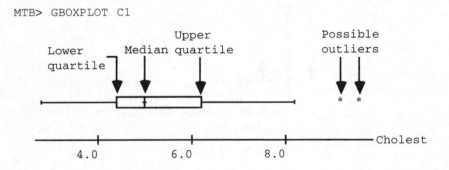

The boxplot displays the main features of the data including the median, the quartiles and possible outliers. The lower whisker gives the (lower quartile) − 1.5 × (the interquartile range). The upper whisker gives the (upper quartile) + 1.5 × (the interquartile range).

1.12   What to watch out for

- Use of the standard deviation to describe non-symmetrical data can lead to nonsensical statements. For example, to describe the mean age of a paediatric population as 5 ± 8 (SD) is clearly inappropriate as this gives the impression that negative ages are possible. The range, median and interquartile range are more meaningful descriptions of such skewed data.
- Precise quantitative statements can be made about the distributions of subjects or units in a population *only* if the distributions are known. For example, if we know that a population is normally distributed with a mean age of 25 ± 5 (SD),

then we can say that approximately 95% of the population is between 15 and 35 years of age.

- The standard deviation and the standard error of the mean (SEM) are commonly reported in the literature without indication as to which is meant. Thus, statements such as 25 ± 5 can be quite misleading if the descriptor (mean ± standard deviation) or (mean ± SEM) is not given.

Chapter 2
Probability and Probability Distributions

2.1 Objectives

In many studies, measurements are made to estimate one or more parameters of the system under study (e.g. aluminium concentration in reservoir water). Those measurements are subject to error and therefore results vary from experiment to experiment. When reporting results there is, therefore, a need to indicate the range within which new results would be expected to fall if the experiment were repeated. If one were able to do this one would be making progress towards defining whether a particular treatment or intervention (e.g. change in water purifying method) had an effect on the parameter of interest (e.g. mean aluminium concentration). In this chapter single parameter estimation is discussed and the terms *probability* and *probability distributions* are defined. The use of probability distributions to describe data from repeated experiments is described and in particular the normal probability distribution is described since it underpins many of the statistical methods discussed in subsequent chapters.

2.2 Probability and probability distributions

Consider what would be observed if a fair coin were thrown a large number of times and the number of heads counted. The first few results of such a study are shown in Table 2.1.

Table 2.1 Outcomes of the first ten throws of a fair coin.

Throw	Outcome			Cumulative fraction showing head
1st	Head	1/1	i.e.	one head out of one throw
2nd	Tail	1/2		one head out of two throws
3rd	Head	2/3		two heads out of three throws
4th	Head	3/4		three heads out of four throws
5th	Tail	3/5		three heads out of five throws
6th	Head	4/6		four heads out of six throws
7th	Tail	4/7		four heads out of seven throws
8th	Tail	4/8		four heads out of eight throws
9th	Head	5/9		five heads out of nine throws
10th	Head	6/10		six heads out of ten throws

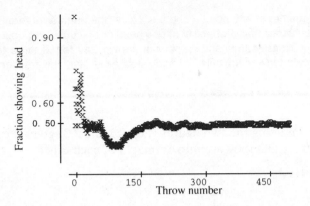

Fig. 2.1 Proportion of throws of a fair coin showing head.

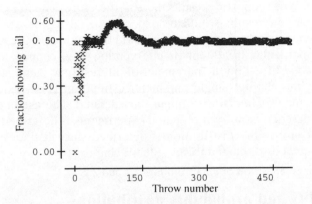

Fig. 2.2 Proportion of throws of a fair coin showing tail.

When the study was pursued further for a total of 500 throws the results shown in Fig. 2.1 were obtained. What is obvious is that the cumulative fraction showing heads settles down to about 0.5. This limiting value is what is known as the *probability* of obtaining a head with the toss of a coin. It is of course generally known that for a fair coin, this probability is equal to 0.5.

Q2.1
If tails were counted instead, what profile would you expect the plot corresponding to Fig. 2.1 to have?

A2.1
The fraction–cumulative count profile would be as shown in Fig. 2.2 except that the probability values would now range from 0 to about 0.5. The simple reason for this is that for any single throw there are only two outcomes, head or tail. Therefore, when we add the two fractions (or

probabilities) together at any point along the *x* axis (the number of throws axis), the sum must equal 1. In other words, the probability of one head or one tail being observed in any one throw is 1 (certainty). Similarly after any number of throws, say ten, if three tails are observed, the fraction of throws turning up tails, is calculated as $\frac{3}{10}$ and the fraction turning up heads is $(1 - \frac{3}{10})$ or $\frac{7}{10}$.

Superimposing the two figures (Figs 2.1 and 2.2) gives the profile shown in Fig. 2.3 showing that they are mirror images of each other.

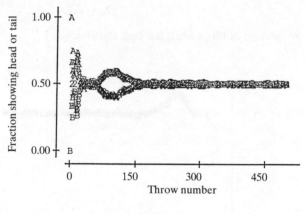

A = Head   B = Tail

Fig. 2.3   Superimposition of data from Figs 2.1 and 2.2.

The figures illustrate two important statistical concepts which are worth reiterating.

(1)   The relative frequency of an event approaches a limiting value as the number of random trials approaches infinity. That limiting value is what is called *probability*. In our coin tossing experiment for any one random trial (a throw) the probability of obtaining a head is said to be 0.5, assuming the coin is fair. This does not mean that one will necessarily obtain one head in two throws as Fig. 2.1 clearly shows.

(2)   Constructing a histogram of the two probabilities, using the limiting values gives Fig. 2.4.

   Such a figure is called a *probability distribution*. It defines the probability of each possible outcome for the process being studied. Given this, the sum of the probabilities of all the individual mutually exclusive outcomes (two in this case) is equal to unity.

A trial such as the one we have just discussed with only two possible outcomes is called a *Bernoulli trial*.

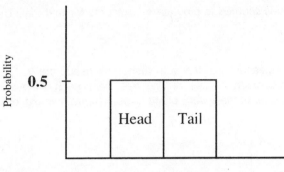

Fig. 2.4 Diagrammatic representation of probability.

Q2.2
What would be the probability distribution for the outcomes associated with the throw of a fair six-sided dice?

A2.2
In this case there are six possible outcomes:

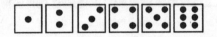

If the dice is thrown an infinitely large number of times we would expect to observe each of those outcomes *on average* once in six throws. Therefore the probability distribution, which gives the probabilities for each possible outcome, is as shown in Fig. 2.5.

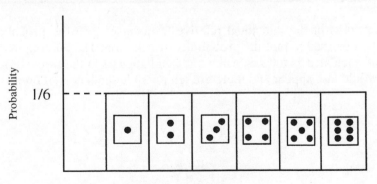

Fig. 2.5 Probability of each possible outcome on the throw of a fair six-sided dice.

Q2.3
Going back to the coin tossing study. What would be the probability distribution for the number of heads in the following experiment? Each trial consists of ten dice being thrown at once and

the number of heads counted to produce an outcome for that trial. The trial is then repeated many times.

A2.3

The possible outcomes for each trial with respect to heads are 0, 1, 2, 3, 4, 5, 6, 7, 8, 9, 10 successes. If the proportion of times (*relative frequency*) each of those outcomes was observed after an infinite number of trials were plotted, the histogram would look like Fig. 2.6.

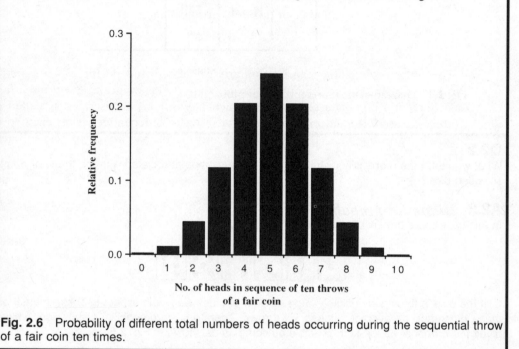

Fig. 2.6 Probability of different total numbers of heads occurring during the sequential throw of a fair coin ten times.

The limits of the individual relative frequencies give the probabilities which can then be used to plot the probability distribution. The limiting frequencies are in fact calculated as follows: when one head appears in the throw of ten dice nine tails would also appear and there are ten possible sequences of one head and nine tails:

```
H T T T T T T T T T
T H T T T T T T T T
T T H T T T T T T T
T T T H T T T T T T
T T T T H T T T T T
T T T T T H T T T T
T T T T T T H T T T
T T T T T T T H T T
T T T T T T T T H T
T T T T T T T T T H
```

Hence the probability of obtaining one head with ten dice is given by:

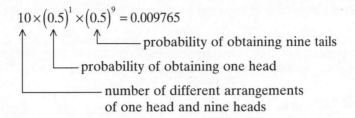

$$10 \times (0.5)^1 \times (0.5)^9 = 0.009765$$

— probability of obtaining nine tails

— probability of obtaining one head

— number of different arrangements of one head and nine heads

The other probabilities can be similarly calculated. Indeed there is a general formula known as the binomial theorem for calculating those probabilities (see Section 2.2.1). The experiment which has just been described is called a *Binomial experiment* since it consists of a series of independent trials each with precisely two outcomes (Bernoulli trials) and the probability of success in each trial is the same.

2.2.1   *Binomial probability*

In a binomial experiment consisting of n trials, each having exactly two outcomes (success or failure) and with a probability of success of p, the probability $p(x)$ of obtaining exactly x successes in n trials is given by:

$$p(x) = \binom{n}{x} p^x (1-p)^{n-x}$$

where

$$\binom{n}{x} = \frac{n(n-1)(n-2)(n-3) \dots (n-x+1)}{x(x-1)(x-2)(x-3) \dots (3)(2)(1)}$$

For example, if the binomial experiment consists of ten tosses of a coin (ten trials), each trial will have two outcomes (heads or tails). The probability of success (e.g. a head) in each trial is p. For a fair coin this is 0.5. The probability $p(x)$ of obtaining exactly x successes (e.g. two heads) in the ten trials is given by

$$p(x) = p(2) = \binom{10}{2}(0.5)^2(1-0.5)^{10-2} = \frac{10 \times 9}{2 \times 1} \times (0.5)^2 (1-0.5)^3 = 0.043945$$

Q2.4
Can you calculate the probability of obtaining three heads in the experiment just described?

A2.4

$$p(x) = p(3) = \binom{10}{3}(0.5)^3(1-0.5)^{10-3}$$

$$= \frac{10 \times 9 \times 8}{3 \times 2 \times 1} \times (0.5)^3 \times (1-0.5)^7 = 0.117188$$

Q2.5
Can you calculate the probability of obtaining three heads in the experiment just described but with a biased coin such that the probability of a head in any one throw is 0.4?

A2.5

$$p(x) = p(3) = \binom{10}{3}(0.3)^3(1-0.3)^{10-3} = 0.266828$$

2.2.2 Continuous distributions

So far the discussion of probability distributions has been concerned with experiments in which there is a *finite* number of different outcomes.

2 in the tossing of a single coin.
6 in the throw of a dice.
11 in the binomial experiment involving throwing ten dice and counting heads.

The variables concerned are called *discrete variables* since the number of values they can take is finite.

In many instances the number of potential outcomes is infinite. For example, if we were to measure the heights of adult men, the height of a randomly chosen individual could be 165, 166, 167, ... cm or indeed any value in between, e.g. 166.275 cm. In constructing a histogram of heights there is therefore an infinite number of possible outcomes provided we have the necessary instrument to measure to the precision required. A variable such as height which can take on an infinite number of values is called a *continuous variable*. Figures 2.7(a)–(c) show histograms of the heights of men from one particular population using a cell width of 5 cm and using samples of 25, 250 and 15 000 men.

Q2.6
What can one detect as sample size increases from 25 to 15 000?

A2.6
The histogram (Fig. 2.7) becomes more symmetrical as sample size increases. What can be shown also is that the reproducibility of the shapes of the histogram improves as sample size

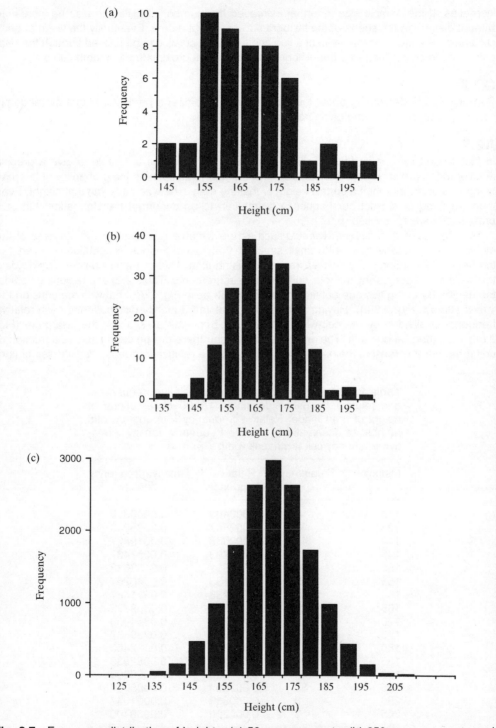

Fig. 2.7 Frequency distribution of heights. (a) 50 measurements, (b) 250 measurements and (c) 15000 measurements.

increases. If the sample size is further increased the number of cells can also be increased without disturbing the shape of the histogram to any great extent. Eventually the width of each cell can be the same as the width of a line and a smooth curve can be passed through the mid-points of the cells. Therefore the histogram eventually approximates a smooth curve.

Q2.7

Can one make statements about the probability of obtaining a particular height by randomly selecting one man from the given population?

A2.7

In fact given that one is dealing with a continuous variable one is unable to give a precise answer to the question posed. Instead we make statements such as the probability of the man being less or greater than a certain height or that the man is between this and that height. Even then we need to subject our frequency distribution to an important transformation that of a *probability density function* (p.d.f.).

As in the case of a *discrete variable* such as the variable representing the outcome of the throw of a dice, one can, with small samples from a continuous distribution, convert the frequency distribution into a *relative* frequency distribution. This can easily be done by dividing the number in each cell by the total number of measurements (Table 2.2) and replotting against the height. By doing this one obtains the same graph as in Fig. 2.7(c) but with the units on the y axis altered (Fig. 2.8(a)). Having obtained the relative frequency distribution, if each relative frequency is divided by the cell width (Table 2.2), 5 cm, the area under the histogram (Fig. 2.8(b)) will then be one unit. The area in each cell can therefore be expressed as a fraction of unit area. For this reason, the new distribution is called a relative frequency *density* distribution.

Table 2.2 Converting frequencies to relative frequencies and relative frequency densities. 15 000 observations of height of men made. Relative frequency = frequency/total number of observations; relative frequency density = relative frequency/cell width; cell width = 5 cm.

Midpoint	Frequency	Relative frequency	Relative frequency density
130	6	0.000400	0.0000800
135	40	0.002667	0.0005333
140	149	0.009933	0.0019867
145	431	0.028733	0.0057467
150	1000	0.066667	0.0133333
155	1847	0.123133	0.0246267
160	2636	0.175733	0.0351467
165	2923	0.194867	0.0389733
170	2658	0.177200	0.0354400
175	1796	0.119733	0.0239467
180	918	0.061200	0.0122400
185	397	0.026467	0.0052933
190	150	0.010000	0.0020000
195	38	0.002533	0.0005067
200	8	0.000533	0.0001067
205	3	0.000200	0.0000400

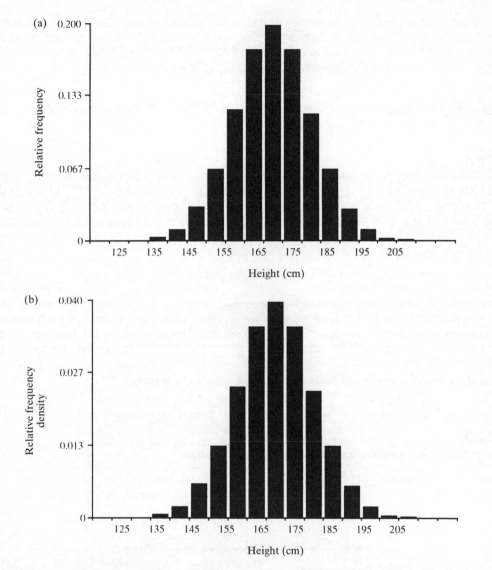

Fig. 2.8   (a) *Relative* frequency distribution of heights and (b) frequency *density* distribution of heights.

As already discussed, if one samples an infinitely large number of men from the population concerned the relative frequency density distribution becomes smoother and smoother until we obtain a smooth curve. At the limit the curve gives the probability density function (Fig. 2.9).

Q2.8
Why should statisticians go to such trouble to construct a probability density function?

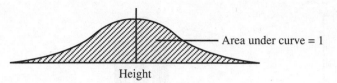
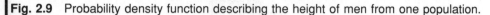

Fig. 2.9 Probability density function describing the height of men from one population.

A2.8

When constructing the probability density function, the frequency density rather than frequency or relative frequency is the ordinate to give an area under the curve which is equal to unit area.

Therefore if one is able to calculate the area under the probability density function curve say between x_1 and x_2 as in Fig. 2.10, one would be able to say that the area gives the probability that a man randomly chosen from the population whose men have heights described by the probability density function shown is between x_1 and x_2.

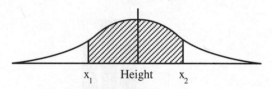
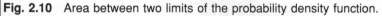

Fig. 2.10 Area between two limits of the probability density function.

Q2.9

What probability does the area shown in Fig. 2.11 describe?

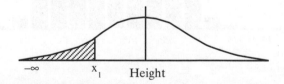

Fig. 2.11 Lower tail of a probability density function.

A2.9

This gives the probability that the height of a man chosen from the population whose men have heights described by the probability density function shown is smaller or equal to x_1. The infinity lower bound is of course meaningless.

Q2.10

What probability does the shaded area shown in Fig. 2.12 describe?

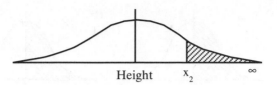

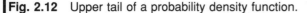

Height x_2 ∞

Fig. 2.12   Upper tail of a probability density function.

A2.10

This gives the probability that the height of a man chosen at random from the population whose men have heights described by the probability density function shown is greater than x_2.

You may be wondering at this stage how we are able to calculate the areas shown. Areas under a curve can be calculated by integrating the equation describing the curve between the limits we are interested in (e.g. x_1 and x_2 or $-\infty$ to x_1). Therefore our first task is to obtain such an equation. Luckily the general bell shape shown in Figs 2.9–2.11 is quite often seen with the distributions of *continuous variables* such as height, weight, length of human pregnancies, random error in physical measurements, etc. Therefore, if we are able to obtain a general equation describing those curves we would be making important progress. The famous mathematician Gauss (1777–1855) in fact developed such an equation which was named in his honour as the equation for the Gaussian distribution. More commonly this equation is now known as the equation for the *normal distribution*.

Standardising a normal distribution

Given a probability density function (e.g. Fig. 2.12), the previous discussion has shown that probability statements about the variable concerned can be made by calculating areas under appropriate sections of the curve by integration. One of the difficulties with this is that the integration is often difficult. It would, therefore, be useful practically if suitable tables of areas under different sections of the different probability density function curves were made available to us. The difficulty is that there is an infinite number of possible probability density curves even for a given type of distribution (e.g. normal distribution) and in practice most statistical tables compile only the more common distributions.

For the normal distribution, it is possible to standardise any of the probability density curves to a standard normal variate which has a mean of 0 and unit standard deviation. This variate is called the **Z** variate. The practical benefit of this is that a single table of areas can be used to calculate specific probabilities.

To understand why this approach works consider the two distributions shown in Fig. 2.13. They are both probability density functions. So, the area under each curve is unity. Curve (a), however, has a mean of 0 and is known as the *standard normal probability density curve*. Curve (b) on the other hand is shifted to the right of (a) and has a mean of 14. The scales used in the two figures are identical.

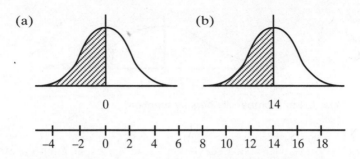

Fig. 2.13 Probability density functions for normally distributed variables: (a) with mean 0 and standard deviation 1 and (b) with mean 14 and standard deviation 1.

It is easy to see that the area from minus infinity to the mean is in each case equal to 0.5 of unity, that is half the total area under each curve. If 14 is taken away from the x coordinate of each point on curve (b) and the values replotted a curve which is superimposable on curve (a) is produced. In other words, the probability density function for a variate with a mean of 14 has been transformed to one with a mean of 0.

Consider now the two figures shown in Fig. 2.14(a) and (b). Figure 2.14(a) represents the probability density curve for the standard normal variate. Figure 2.14(b) is the probability density function for a normally distributed variable also with a mean of 0 but with a standard deviation of 0.8. Again, the shaded area in each figure is equal to 0.5 of unity since the curves are symmetrical and the shaded area is half the total area in each case. If each x value in Fig. 2.14(b) is divided by 0.8 and the values replotted a curve superimposable on Fig. 2.14(a) is obtained. In other words the variate with standard deviation 0.8 had been standardised to the standard normal variate with standard deviation 1.

A normal variate can of course be standardised both with respect to its mean and to its standard deviation. To do this the mean is taken away from each x value

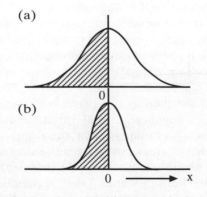

Fig. 2.14 Probability density functions for (a) the standard normal variate and (b) for a normally distributed variable with mean 0 and standard deviation 0.8.

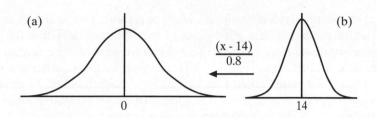

Fig. 2.15 Standardising a normal distribution with mean 14 and standard deviation 0.8. (a) Standard normal distribution, that is with mean 0 and standard deviation 1 and (b) normal distribution with mean 14 and standard deviation 0.8.

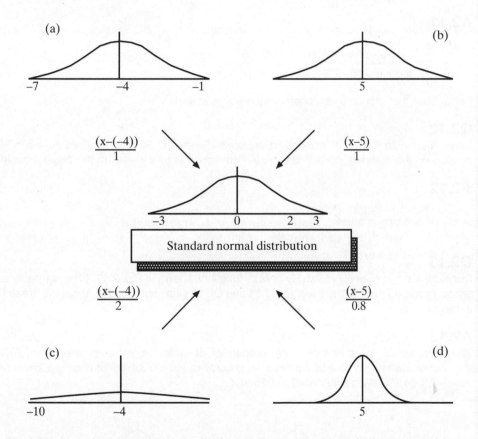

Fig. 2.16 Transforming normal distributions to the *standard* normal distribution. (a) Normal distribution with mean −4 and standard deviation 1; (b) normal distribution with mean 5 and standard deviation 1; (c) normal distribution with mean −4 and standard deviation 2 and (d) normal distribution with mean 5 and standard deviation 0.8.

and the result divided by the standard deviation. This is shown in Fig. 2.15 for a standard normal variate with mean 14 and standard deviation 0.8.

Standardisation as just described therefore enables one to find a point on the standard normal curve (Fig. 2.15(a)) corresponding to another one on the distribution being standardised (e.g. in Fig. 2.15 the point labelled 14 in curve (b) corresponds to point 0 on curve (a). Figure 2.16 shows standardisation of some other distributions to the standard normal distribution.

Q2.11

Given a variable (x) which is normally distributed with mean 50 and variance 16, what value (z) on the standard normal distribution corresponds to $x = 20$ in the original distribution?

A2.11

$$z = \frac{20 - (\text{mean of } x)}{\text{standard deviation of } x} = \frac{20 - 50}{\sqrt{16}} = -7.5$$

Remember that standard deviation = square root of variance.

Q2.12

Given a variable X which is normally distributed with mean -30 and standard deviation 5, what z-value on the standard normal distribution corresponds to $x = -10$ on the original curve?

A2.12

$$z = \frac{-10 - (-30)}{5} = 4$$

Q2.13

Consider the two normal probability density functions shown in Fig. 2.17. (The diagrams are not drawn to scale.) From the answer to Q2.11 and Q2.12 what can one say about the areas shown in the two figures?

A2.13

They are equal. In other words the probability of finding a value smaller than 20 in the distribution with mean 50 and variance 16 is equal to the probability of finding a value smaller than -7.5 on the standard normal distribution.

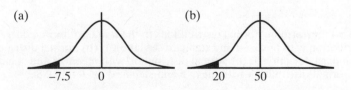

Fig. 2.17 Graphs for Question 2.11 showing (a) mean 0 and standard deviation 1 and (b) mean 50 and variance 16.

Q2.14
Consider the two normal probability density functions shown in Fig. 2.18 (not drawn to scale). From the answer in Q2.11 and Q2.12 what can one say about the areas to the left of 4 and −10 in the two distributions?

A2.14
They are both equal. Hence the probability of finding a value smaller than −10 in the distribution shown on the right is the same as the probability of obtaining a value smaller than 4 in the distribution shown in the figure on the left of Fig. 2.18.

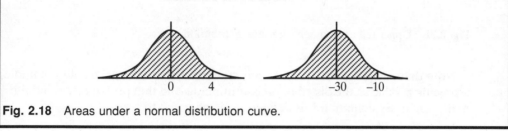

Fig. 2.18   Areas under a normal distribution curve.

From the discussion it should be clear that probability statements can be made about any variable with a normal distribution by reference to the standard normal variate. The types of probability statements which can be made are:

(1) the probability of finding a value smaller or equal to a given value (z). This is given by the area from $-\infty$ to that value under the standard normal density curve (Fig. 2.19).

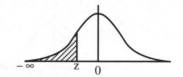
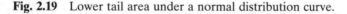

Fig. 2.19   Lower tail area under a normal distribution curve.

(2) the probability of finding a value between two z-values, z_1 and z_2. This is given by the area shown in Fig. 2.20.

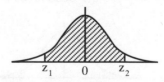
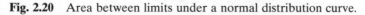

Fig. 2.20   Area between limits under a normal distribution curve.

(3)   the probability of finding a value greater than z_1. This is given by the area *above* z_1. This is equivalent to 1 minus the area *below* z_1. Remember that since the figure is that of a probability *density* function the total area under the curve = 1 (Fig. 2.21).

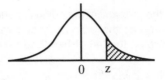

Fig. 2.21   Upper tail area under a normal distribution curve.

Note that one is not able to make any statement about the probability of finding a specific z-value as the distribution is continuous and that probability is infinitesimally small. By definition it is defined as being equal to zero.

Finding the area below a z-value

What is needed is a way of obtaining areas below or above specific z-values. In other words integration of the standard probability density function between appropriate limits is required. This can be done quite easily by computer or more tediously by calculator.

In practice one does not need to do this since appropriate tables are readily available. One such table is given in Appendix 1 which lists areas to the right of specific z-values (Fig. 2.22). You can therefore read that the area above a z-value of 1.96 is 0.025. Neave (1979) also provides detailed statistical tables.

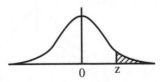

Fig. 2.22   Upper tail area of the standard normal curve.

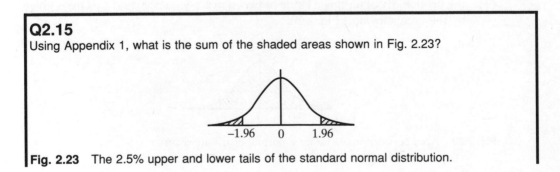

Q2.15

Using Appendix 1, what is the sum of the shaded areas shown in Fig. 2.23?

Fig. 2.23   The 2.5% upper and lower tails of the standard normal distribution.

A2.15

The area = (area above $z = 1.96$) + (area below $z = -1.96$)

$$= 0.025 + 0.025 = 0.05.$$

Q2.16

What is the area (a) above $z = 1.64$ and (b) above $z = 1.64$ and below $z = -1.64$.

A2.16

(a)   0.05
(b)   0.05 + 0.05 = 0.10.

Q2.17

What is the area (a) above $z = 2.58$, (b) above $z = 2.58$ and below $z = -2.58$, (c) above $z = 3.29$ and (d) above $z = 3.29$ and below $z = -3.29$.

A2.17

(a)   0.005
(b)   0.005 + 0.005 = 0.010
(c)   0.0005
(d)   0.0005 + 0.0005 = 0.001.

Q2.18 an extended question

A headache tablet manufacturer produces paracetamol tablets whose drug content is labelled 500 mg. Suppose that the weights are in fact normally distributed with a mean of 502 mg and a variance of 50 mg^2.

(a)   What proportion of the tablets contain less than 500 mg?
(b)   What proportion of the tablets contain less than 490 or more than 510 mg of paracetamol?
(c)   What proportion of the tablets contain more than 520 mg?
(d)   A customer buys a pack of 25 tablets from this batch of tablets. What is the probability that at most 1 tablet contains less than 490 mg?

A2.18(a)

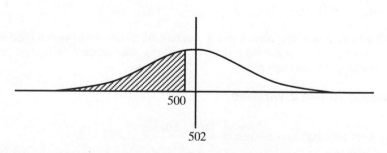

Fig. 2.24   A sketch of the probability density function for the paracetamol content of the tablets.

Standardising

$$z = \frac{500 - 502}{\sqrt{50}}$$

i.e. $\dfrac{[500 - (\text{population})]}{\text{standard deviation of population}}$

$$= -0.283$$

Looking up a probability value

The probability of the z-value being lower than -0.283 (obtained from the table of values of probabilities in the normal distribution given in Neave (1979) = 0.3885. This probability is shown by the shaded region relative to the whole area under the curve (Fig. 2.24).

Hence the proportion of tablets containing less than 500 mg paracetamol is 0.3885.

A2.18(b)

The proportion of tablets containing less than 490 mg, given that the paracetamol content of the tablets is normally distributed with variance 50 mg², is given by area α_1 in Fig. 2.25(a) and (c).

The proportion of tablets with a paracetamol content below 510 mg is given by area α_2 in Fig. 2.25(b).

(a)   (b)

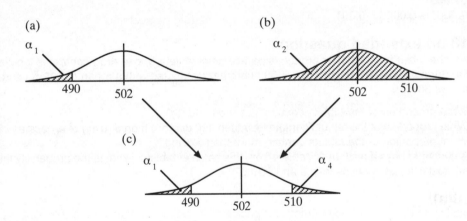

(c)

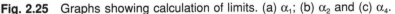

Fig. 2.25 Graphs showing calculation of limits. (a) α_1; (b) α_2 and (c) α_4.

The proportion of tablets with a paracetamol content below 490 mg or above 510 mg

$$= \alpha_1 + \alpha_4 = \alpha_1 + (1 - \alpha_2) = 1 + \alpha_1 - \alpha_2$$

Note that the total area under each curve is normalised to unit area; hence area $\alpha_4 = 1 - \alpha_2$. α_4 is not calculated directly since in the probability table for the standard normal distribution only areas below specific z-values are given.

Standardising to the z variable

490 mg corresponds to a z-value of $\dfrac{(490 - 502)}{\sqrt{50}} = -1.697$

510 mg corresponds to a z-value of $\dfrac{(510 - 502)}{\sqrt{50}} = 1.131$

Area α_1 = area below $z = -1.697$ in the z curve = 0.0448.

Area α_2 = area below $z = 1.131$ in the z curve = 0.8710.

Area $\alpha_4 = 1 - \alpha_2 = 1 - 0.8710 = 0.129$.

Area $(\alpha_1 + \alpha_4) = 0.0448 + 0.129 = 0.1738$
$\qquad\qquad$ = probability of proportion of tablets being less than 490 mg or more than 510 mg.

A2.18(c)

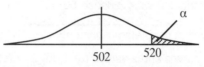

Fig. 2.26   Fraction of tablets containing more than 520 mg paracetamol.

Proportion of tablets containing more than $520 \text{mg} = \dfrac{520 - 502}{\sqrt{50}} = 2.546$

Probability of z being lower than 2.546 in z-distribution = 0.99437.

Probability of z-value being greater than 2.546 = 1 − 0.99437 = 0.00563 = α (Fig. 2.26).

$\therefore$ Proportion of tablets being greater than 520 mg is 0.00563.

A2.18(d)

Probability that *at most* 1 tablet out of the packet of 25 tablets contains more than 520 mg is equal to

P = Probability that no tablet in the packet contains more than 520 mg ($P(x = 0)$)
$\quad$ + Probability that 1 tablet in the packet contains more than 520 mg ($P(x = 1)$).

$P(x = 0)$ = Probability of all 25 tablets containing 520 mg or less of paracetamol
$\qquad\quad = (0.99437)^{25} = 0.868$.

$P(x = 1)$ = Probability of one tablet containing more than 510 mg and all the other 24
$\qquad\quad$ containing 520 mg or less of paracetamol
$\qquad\quad = (25)(0.00563)^1(0.99437)^{24}$
$\qquad\quad = 0.123$.

$\therefore$ $P = 0.868 + 0.123 = 0.991$.

Note that the 25 multiplier is introduced because any one of the 25 tablets could be the one containing more than 520 mg of paracetamol.

Q2.19

Given the standard normal distribution (i.e. mean zero and unit standard deviation) and the table in Appendix 1, calculate the three shaded areas shown in Fig. 2.27.

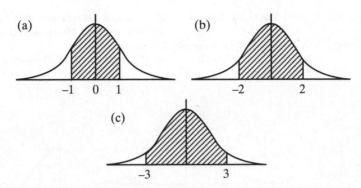

Fig. 2.27   Standard normal curves and z-values (a) 1, (b) 2 or (c) 3 standard deviations from the mean.

A2.19

(a) $(0.5 - 0.1587) \times 2 = 0.6826$ or 68.3% of total area.
(b) $(0.5 - 0.0228) \times 2 = 0.9544$ or 95.4% of total area.
(c) $(0.5 - 0.00135) \times 2 = 0.9973$ or 99.7% of total area.
   Those areas can be expressed as in Fig. 2.28.

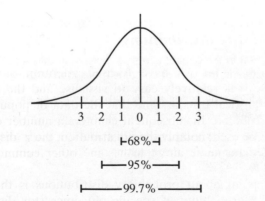

Fig. 2.28   Percentage of data within 1, 2 and 3 standard deviations of the mean of the standard normal distribution.

Q2.20

Consider the normal distribution of heights of men, discussed earlier in this chapter, with mean 165 cm and standard deviation of 10 cm. How many men from that population would have heights between (a) 155 and 175 cm; (b) 145 and 185 cm and (c) 136 and 195 cm?

A2.20

Those limits are within (a) 1 standard deviation, (b) 2 standard deviations and (c) 3 standard deviations of the mean, 165 cm (see Fig. 2.29). Therefore from A2.19 we would expect 68, 95 and 99.7% of men to fall respectively in intervals (a), (b) and (c).

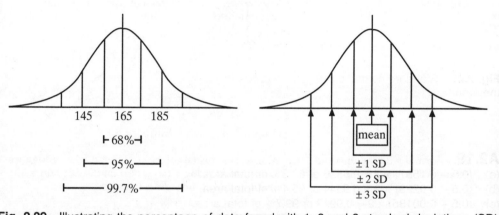

Fig. 2.29 Illustrating the percentage of data found with 1, 2 and 3 standard deviations (SD) from the mean.

2.2.3   Other probability distributions

In the discussion so far we have focused attention on the binomial distribution because it is relatively easy to visualise and the normal distribution because many statistical tests assume that the data or populations under study are normally distributed. In subsequent chapters a number of other probability distributions will be used, notably the t-distribution, the χ^2 distribution and the F-distribution. Their formulae along with some other common distributions are given in Table 2.3.

The essential point about probability distributions is that they enable the calculation of the probability of specific outcomes (for discrete distributions) or the probability of obtaining outcomes in a given range (for continuous distributions).

Table 2.3 Continuous distributions.

Name	Formula for the probability density function (p.d.f.)
Chi-square with ν degrees of freedom	χ^2 distribution with ν degrees of freedom. $$f(x) = \frac{x^{(\nu-2)/2}e^{-x/2}}{2^{\nu/2}\,\Gamma(\nu/2)}, \qquad x > 0, \nu > 0$$
Exponential with parameter $1/b$	Exponential distribution. $$f(x) = \frac{1}{b}e^{-x/b}, \qquad x > 0, b > 0$$
F with u and ν degrees of freedom	F-distribution with u degrees of freedom for the numerator and ν degrees of freedom for the denominator. $$f(x) = \frac{\Gamma[(u+\nu)/2]}{\Gamma[u/2]\Gamma[\nu/2]}\left(\frac{u}{\nu}\right)^{u/2}$$ $$\frac{x^{(u-2)/2}}{\left[1+(u/\nu)x\right]^{(u+\nu)/2}}, \qquad x > 0, u > 0, \nu > 0$$ where Γ is gamma distribution
Lognormal with mean μ and standard deviation σ	Lognormal distribution. A variable x has a lognormal distribution if $\log x$ has a normal distribution with mean μ and standard deviation σ. $$f(x) = \frac{1}{x\sqrt{2\pi}\sigma}e^{-[(\log_e x)-\mu]^2/2\sigma^2}, \qquad x > 0$$
Normal with mean μ and standard deviation σ	Normal distribution with mean ν and standard deviation σ. $$f(x) = \frac{1}{\sqrt{2\pi}\sigma}e^{-(x-\mu)^2/2\sigma^2}, \qquad \sigma > 0$$
t with ν degrees of freedom	Student's t-distribution with ν degrees of freedom. $$f(x)\frac{\Gamma[(\nu+1)/2]}{\Gamma[\nu/2]\sqrt{\nu\pi}}\frac{1}{\left(1+x^2/\nu\right)^{(\nu+1)/2}}, \qquad \nu > 0$$
Uniform with range $[a, b]$	Uniform distribution on a to b. $$f(x) = \frac{1}{b-a}, \qquad a < x < b$$

Chapter 3
Hypothesis Testing

3.1 Objective of a hypothesis test

A statistical hypothesis is a statement about what one believes about the value of one or more population parameters or about the probabilistic mechanism which has generated the observations under consideration. A hypothesis test is a test of that belief. Two examples will help to illustrate these concepts.

3.2 Hypothesis test about population parameters

A quick observation of a population of a particular insect may lead one to believe that the female of the species is larger than the male. This, therefore, forms our hypothesis which can be tested by collecting data on a random sample basis of male and female insects of that species.

3.3 Hypothesis test about probabilistic mechanism

Genetic manipulation to produce plants or animals which have more desirable attributes than existing varieties or species is widely used and much effort has been, and continues to be, directed towards understanding the mechanisms by which particular characteristics are transferred. Mendel in studying the inheritance of genes from several loci hypothesised that the alleles of different genes of an individual divide independently of each other when the gamete is formed and are therefore inherited independently by an offspring. By cross-fertilising peas and recording the characteristic of F_2 peas he was able to test and thereby support his hypothesis now known as Mendel's second law of genetic inheritance.

Although hypothesis testing with respect to population parameters and probabilistic mechanisms may initially appear to be completely different, both involve the same steps shown in Fig. 3.1.

Example 3.1

Suppose that it was not generally known that Swiss boys tended to be taller than girls at age 15 and the hypothesis put forward was that this was the case. Let μ_1 represent the girls' mean height at age 15 and μ_2 the corresponding boys' height. One can therefore proceed with steps 1 and 2 shown in Fig. 3.1.

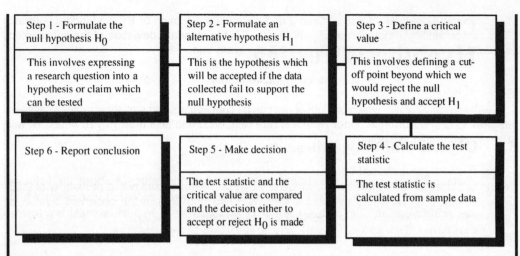

Fig. 3.1   Steps involved in carrying out a hypothesis test.

Solution

Step 1: Formulate the null hypothesis

$$H_0 : \mu_1 = \mu_2 \qquad \text{or} \qquad \mu_2 - \mu_1 = 0$$

The null hypothesis states that the mean heights are equal.

Step 2: Formulate an alternative hypothesis

$$H_1 : \mu_2 > \mu_1 \qquad \text{or} \qquad \mu_2 - \mu_1 > 0$$

The alternative hypothesis is that the mean height of the boys is larger than that of the girls. Note that this was the *original* hypothesis.

To carry out steps 3 and 4 one needs two things: (1) sample data from which we shall be making inferences about our population of boys and girls and (2) some knowledge about the probability distribution of the summary measure (test statistic) one is going to calculate from the sample data. One needs the latter because without it one is unable to make precise statements about how likely or unlikely an observation is. Perhaps analogy to the case of the throw of a dice will clarify this further. Unless one knows that each number on a conventional fair dice has a probability of 1/6 of turning up one is unable to make precise statements about how likely two sixes in a row are.

Statistical theory states that if the variables x_1 and x_2, the boys' and girls' heights, are normally distributed or if the sample sizes n_1 and n_2 taken for estimating the mean heights are large (>30), then the statistic

$$\frac{(\bar{x}_1 - \bar{x}_2) - (\mu_1 - \mu_2)}{s_{\bar{x}_1 - \bar{x}_2}} = z \qquad (3.1)$$

will be normally distributed with a mean 0 and a standard deviation of 1 (i.e. standard normal). This can be written in notation as $Z \sim N(0, 1^2)$. S is the standard deviation of the subscripted variable. Since H_0 postulates that $\mu_1 - \mu_2 = 0$, if it were true

$$(\bar{x}_1 - \bar{x}_2)/s_{\bar{x}_1 - \bar{x}_2}$$ will also be standard normal.

Therefore any z-value which one observes can be checked against statistical tables to assess its likelihood of occurrence under H_0. If it is rare (e.g. occurring less than 1 in 20 times) H_0 will be rejected and H_1 accepted.

Step 3: Defining a critical value
With the standard normal variate, a z-value of 1.645 or greater occurs with a probability of 0.05 (see Appendix 1). Therefore the critical value is 1.645 (Fig. 3.2). If the observed z-value is greater than this value, H_0 will be rejected and H_1 accepted.

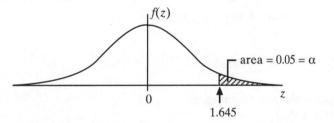

Fig. 3.2   Probability density function for $(\bar{x}_1 - \bar{x}_2)/s_{\bar{x}_1 - \bar{x}_2}$ or z.

Table 3.1   Heights of random samples of 15-year-old Swiss boys and girls (arranged in ascending order for convenience).

Boys (cm):	152.4, 155.7, 157.9, 158.8, 159.0, 161.0, 161.0, 162.8, 163.0, 164.2, 164.6, 165.1, 165.2, 165.5, 166.1, 166.2, 167.1, 167.5, 167.8, 170.4, 170.7, 170.7, 171.1, 172.1, 173.4, 173.9, 174.4, 176.9, 177.7, 180.9
Girls (cm):	153.6, 153.9, 155.3, 156.0, 156.2, 156.9, 156.9, 157.0, 157.6, 157.7, 157.7, 158.7, 159.7, 160.4, 160.8, 160.9, 162.9, 163.3, 163.3, 163.7, 164.1, 164.4, 165.0, 165.1, 166.5, 167.8, 168.1, 168.3, 169.8, 170.6

Step 4: Calculate the test statistic
To illustrate step 4 consider the data in Table 3.1 which shows the heights of random samples of Swiss boys and girls. The statistic can be calculated to be 3.52 as shown below.

Step by step calculation of the test statistic
$\bar{x}_1$ = mean height of the boys
    $= (152.4 + 155.7 + \ldots + 177.7 + 180.9)/30 = 166.77$

s_{x_1} = standard deviation of the boys' heights

$$= \sqrt{\frac{(152.4 - 166.77)^2 + (155.7 - 166.7)^2 + \ldots + (180.9 - 166.7)^2}{(30 - 1)}} = 6.73$$

$\bar{x}_2$ = mean height of the girls
$$= (153.6 + 153.9 + \ldots + 169.8 + 170.6)/30 = 161.41$$

s_{x_2} = standard deviation of the girls' heights

$$= \sqrt{\frac{(153.6 - 161.41)^2 + (153.9 - 161.41)^2 + \ldots + (170.6 - 161.41)^2}{(30 - 1)}} = 4.90$$

To calculate our test statistic z we need the standard deviation of $(\bar{x}_1 - \bar{x}_2)$ or $s_{\bar{x}_1 - \bar{x}_2}$. If we assume that both population heights (boys and girls) have the same standard deviation σ then σ, the *pooled standard deviation*, can be estimated using the formula

$$\sigma = \sqrt{\frac{(n_1 - 1)s_1^2 + (n_2 - 1)s_2^2}{n_1 + n_2 - 2}}$$

In our case $n_1 = n_2 = 30$, the sample sizes of the boys and girls respectively. Therefore

$$\sigma = \sqrt{\frac{29 \times 6.73^2 + 29 \times 4.90^2}{60 - 2}} = 5.89$$

The *test statistic* is therefore given by

$$z = \frac{(\bar{x}_1 - \bar{x}_2)}{\sigma \sqrt{(1/n_1 + 1/n_2)}} \qquad = 3.52$$

$$= \frac{(166.77 - 161.41)}{5.89 \sqrt{(1/30 + 1/30)}} \qquad = 3.52$$

Step 5: Make decision
Since a value of $z = 1.645$ or greater occurs only 1 in 20 times under H_0 then a value of 3.52 or greater occurs even more rarely; in fact with a probability of 0.000193. Therefore H_0 is rejected and H_1 accepted.

Step 6: Report conclusions
The data strongly indicate that the mean boys' height at 15 years of age is higher than that of the corresponding girls' height.

3.4   Questions about hypothesis testing

3.4.1   *Choosing a hypothesis test*

In the preceding discussion the z statistic was used in order to make precise probability statements about the observed difference in mean sample heights of the boys and girls by reference to a table of probabilities in the normal distribution. How do we choose the test statistic and the probability distribution in other cases? Fortunately many statisticians have addressed this question and useful guidelines can be given for specific types of hypothesis tests. Indeed in the subsequent chapters those guidelines are highlighted. For now it is perhaps sufficient to note that the probability distribution of the possible statistics can often be worked out by recourse to what is known about the distributions of other variables. When this is not possible, simulation techniques can be used to derive the appropriate probability distributions. This approach is commonly used to confirm theoretically derived probability distributions.

3.4.2   Choosing a level of significance (α)

The α-level of a hypothesis test defines the strength of evidence which is deemed to be sufficient for rejection of the null hypothesis (H_0). Often, an α-level of 0.05 or an observation which has a probability of occurring only 1 in 20 times under H_0 is chosen as the cut-off point for rejection of H_0. There is nothing immutable about this α-level of 0.05. It is simply a convention initiated by Sir R.A. Fisher, one of the pioneers of modern statistics. Indeed the α-level should be chosen based on the importance of the decision being made and the consequences of falsely accepting or rejecting H_0. For example, if rejection of a null hypothesis means introduction of a much more expensive treatment or a much more elaborate test procedure, then very few people would be convinced by a significance level of 0.05.

3.4.3   Why define an α-level at all?

Defining an α-level provides an objective way for testing a hypothesis. If the aim of a study is purely to obtain evidence in support of or against a given hypothesis then calculating the appropriate P-value and examining the confidence interval would be more useful than arbitrarily assigning an α-value. However, in applications such as quality control test procedures of products using predefined protocols, a predefined α-level ensures consistency across laboratories, countries, etc., in the way *decisions* are made about rejection or acceptance of the same hypothesis (e.g. about the quality of a product). Examination of crude data for outliers would, however, still be essential.

3.4.4   Statistical versus practical significance

Rejection of the null hypothesis at the usual α-levels (0.05, 0.01 or 0.001) means that there is good evidence of an effect, with the evidence strengthening as the α-level decreases. However rejection of H_0 does not by itself indicate that there is a practically or clinically important effect. Very small effects of no practical value will show up as statistically significant if large samples are used. Therefore when evaluating experimental data it is useful to avoid focusing too much on the α-value. It is good practice to calculate the P value (i.e. the probability of occurrence of the observed value for the parameter of interest under H_0) and to examine appropriate plots of the data particularly for *outliers* which may lead to false conclusions. It is also useful to give a confidence interval for the parameter of interest since instead of simply defining whether an effect is too large to occur by chance alone as does a hypothesis test, it gives an estimate of the size of the effect. The calculation of confidence intervals, power of a test and sample sizes are discussed in Chapter 11.

Chapter 4
Hypothesis Testing About a Single Population Parameter or Paired Data

4.1 Hypothesis testing about a single population parameter

A *parameter* is any measure which describes a population. Examples of population parameters are the mean (μ), the proportion with a given characteristic (π) and the variance (σ^2). Very often one wishes to make inferences about those parameters using samples drawn from populations. Using the samples, corresponding measures are calculated. Such sample measures are called *statistics*. The sample mean ($\bar{x}$), the sample proportion with a given characteristic (p) and the sample variance (s^2) are commonly used statistics. This chapter describes the choice of appropriate hypothesis tests for making inferences about population parameters.

In many studies a single group of subjects is studied under two separate experimental conditions to make use of the fact that inter-subject variability in the response, or in factors which may affect the response, is smaller than intra-subject variability. For example, the data may be measures of food intake before and after a health education session. Therefore each subject provides a pair of measurements. While this study design, sometimes called *within-subject* design, eliminates one problem, namely inter-subject variability, it introduces another, that is, correlation between the measurements.

Such data are often analysed by the usual single sample methods. The difference between each pair of measurements is first calculated and the resulting set of differences is treated as a single data set.

The appropriate hypothesis test will depend on a number of features relating to the samples being investigated and the type of data being collected. Two of the most important considerations are the sample sizes and whether the samples come from populations which follow known distributions and in particular the normal distribution. If one were to take samples from a given population or populations and calculate a suitable statistic such as the mean from each sample, one could construct a probability distribution for that statistic. For the sample mean this can be done by plotting the probability with which the different sample means occur when many samples are drawn. The probability distribution of the sample statistic is known as the *sampling distribution*. If the sampling distribution can be described by one of the known probability distributions (e.g. normal distribution, *t*-distribution or *F*-distribution), then the hypothesis test can be based on the *parameters* of the distribution concerned. Such tests are referred to as *parametric tests* as already discussed.

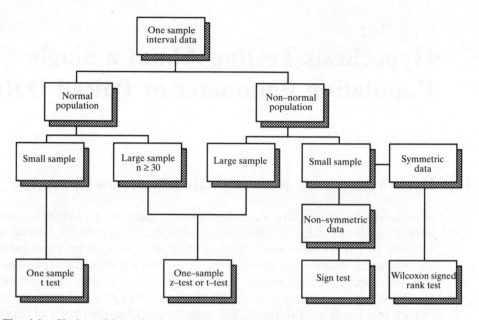

Fig. 4.1 Choice of hypothesis test for making inferences about a population mean or median.

In most textbooks parametric and non-parametric tests are considered separately. In the present presentation both types of tests are considered concurrently to mirror, more closely, practical decision making. Figure 4.1 shows a flow diagram for choosing an appropriate hypothesis test for making inferences about a population mean or about the mean difference for paired data.

4.2 The Z-test – one sample

4.2.1 Background

Assumptions about the data:

Sample is drawn from a distribution with mean, μ, and variance, σ^2

Therefore, if sample n is large ($n > 30$), the sample mean ($\bar{x}$) will be normally distributed with mean μ and variance σ^2/n

$$\bar{x} \sim N\left(\mu, \sigma^2/n\right) \tag{4.1}$$

4.2.2 Mechanics of the test

Step 1
Set up the null and alternative hypotheses.

$H_0: \mu = k$
$H_1: \mu \neq k$

where k is some constant

Step 2
Calculate z-value (i.e. standardise).

Standardising gives

$$z = \frac{\bar{x} - k}{\sqrt{(\sigma^2/n)}} \qquad (4.2)$$

Approximating, as n is large, gives

$$z = \frac{\bar{x} - k}{\sqrt{(s^2/n)}} \sim N(0,\ 1) \qquad (4.3)$$

Note that s^2/n is the variance of the sampling distribution of $\bar{x}$. The square root of this term is called the standard error. H_0 is rejected if z is sufficiently far from 0.

Step 3
Compare z-value against the critical value tabulated in Appendix 1.

The critical region is shown by the shaded area. If the calculated Z statistic falls in this region, then H_0 is rejected. The critical value, z_c, is obtained from statistical tables. Thus, at the 5% significance level, $z_c = 1.96$ (see Appendix 1 and Table 4.1).

Table 4.1 Commonly used Z critical values.

Critical z_c value	Two-sided test α	One-sided test α
1.28	0.2	0.10
1.645	0.1	0.05
1.96	0.05	0.025
2.33	0.02	0.01
2.58	0.01	0.005
3.09	0.02	0.001
3.29	0.001	0.0005

What the 5% significance level means is that, if the curve under the standard normal probability function is integrated from $z = 1.96$ to infinity, then the area will equal 0.025 or 2.5% of the total area. In other words (see Fig. 4.2)

$$P(|z| \geq 1.96) = 0.05$$

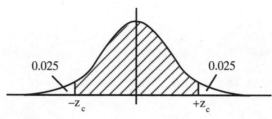

Fig. 4.2 Critical z-values.

Values extreme enough to give z-values in the critical region will only occur 5% of the time if H_0 holds.

Step 4
Draw appropriate conclusion.

Example 4.1

During the manufacture of a 1 litre infusion, 50 bottles were drawn at random and the volume of each container measured to check whether the full volume met the 1 litre claim.

The mean volume, $\bar{x}$, was found to be 1008 ml and the standard deviation was 65 ml. Is there sufficient evidence to suggest that the average volume of the infusion was not 1 litre?

Solution

Step 1
    $H_0 : \mu = 1000\,\text{ml}$
    $H_1 : \mu \neq 1000\,\text{ml}$

Step 2
$$z = \frac{1008 - 1000}{65/\sqrt{50}} = 0.870$$

Step 3
This z-value is not in the critical region as z_c, at a significance probability of 0.05, is 1.96 for a two-sided test (Fig. 4.3).

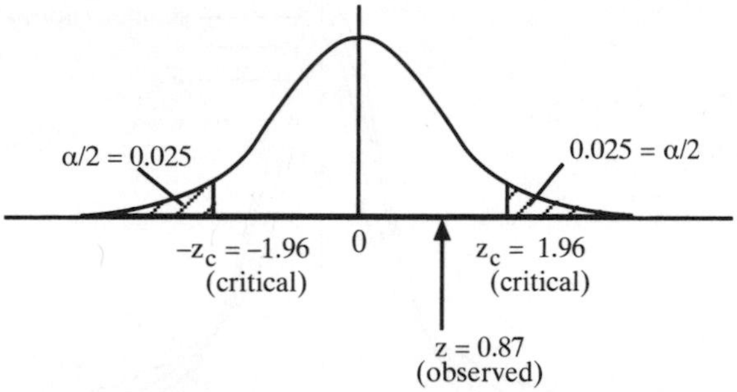

Fig. 4.3 Two-sided Z-test at a significance probability of 0.05.

Step 4

There is, therefore, insufficient evidence to suggest that the full volume was not 1000 ml.

Note: For a one-sided test, the alternative hypothesis would have been either $H_1 : \mu > 1000$ ml or $H_1 : \mu < 1000$ ml. The z_c value at the 0.05 significance probability would now be 1.645 instead of 1.96 (Fig. 4.4). The appropriate values are shown in Table 4.1.

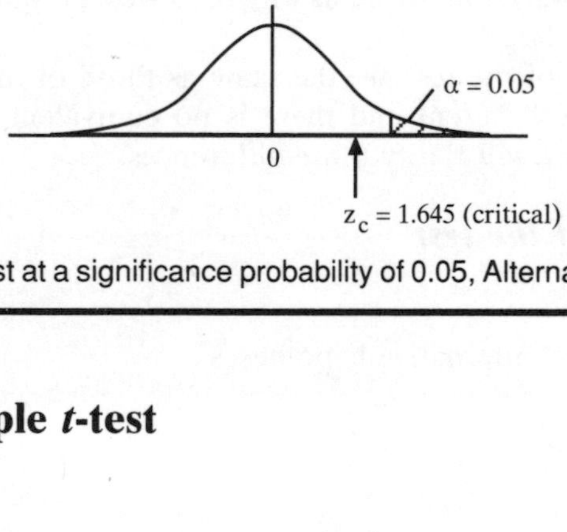

Fig. 4.4   One-sided Z-test at a significance probability of 0.05, Alternative hypothesis $H_1 : \mu > k_0$.

4.3   The one sample *t*-test

4.3.1   *Background*

Often, the variance of the characteristic under study in the population concerned is not known and is estimated from the sample. By so doing another source of unreliability in our data is introduced. This additional unreliability is significant with small sample sizes ($n < 30$). Therefore when probability statements are made about specific outcomes under those conditions, one is no longer justified in using the standard normal distribution even if the underlying population is normally distributed. One statistician, Gosset, using the pen-name 'Student', showed that the sample means under those conditions in fact followed distributions now called Student's *t*-distributions, in his honour. The *t*-distributions are somewhat broader than the corresponding normal distributions as shown in Fig. 4.5. As the sample size increases the *t*-distribution gets closer and closer to the corresponding normal

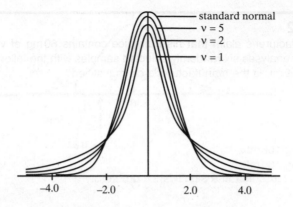

Fig. 4.5 Comparison of the standard normal distribution with the t-distribution with varying degrees of freedom.

distribution (Fig. 4.5). This explains why the Z-test is equivalent to the t-test when the sample size is large.

The mechanics of the test are the same as those of the Z-test except that the critical values are different and there is no equivalent to the *standard* normal curve. Example 4.2 will clarify those differences.

4.3.2 Mechanics of the test

Step 1
Set up the null and alternative hypotheses.

$$H_0 : \mu = k$$
$$H_1 : \mu \neq k$$

Step 2
Calculate t statistic.

$$t = \frac{\bar{x} - \mu}{s} \tag{4.4}$$

Step 3
Compare test statistic against critical value from the t-distribution with $(n - 1)$ degrees of freedom where n is the sample size.

Step 4
Draw appropriate conclusion.

Example 4.2

To test a manufacturer's claim that his fruit juice contains 60 mg of vitamin C per 100 ml, a quality controller analyses six randomly selected samples with the following results: 65, 58, 62, 57, 62, 65 mg/100 ml. Is the manufacturer's claim justified?

Solution

Step 1

$H_0 : \mu = 60$ mg/100 ml

$H_1 : \mu \neq 60$ mg/100 ml

Step 2

$$t = \frac{\bar{x} - \mu}{s}$$

Since $\bar{x} = \dfrac{65 + 58 + 62 + 57 + 62 + 65}{6}$

$= 61.5$

and $s = \left[(65 - 61.5)^2 + (58 - 61.5)^2 + (62 - 61.5)^2 + (57 - 61.5)^2 + (62 - 61.5)^2 \right.$

$\left. + (65 - 61.5)^2 \right] / (6 - 1)$

$= 3.391$

Step 3

Compare against critical value. Since the alternative hypothesis calls for a two-sided test, the *t*-statistic must be compared against a critical value for such a test. This comes from the *t*-distribution with $(n - 1)$ or 5 degrees of freedom. At a significance probability α of 0.05, the critical value $t_c = 2.571$. Therefore, since the test statistic *t* is 1.08 (Table 4.2) and hence smaller than t_c, we have no reason to reject H_0.

Table 4.2 Selected critical values for the *t*-test.

	Two–sided test		One–sided test	
Significance probability (α)	0.01	0.05	0.01	0.05
Degrees of freedom				
1	63.657	12.706	31.821	6.314
2	9.925	4.303	6.965	2.920
3	5.841	3.182	4.541	2.353
4	4.604	2.776	3.747	2.132
5	4.032	2.571	3.365	2.015

Step 4
The manufacturer's claim that his fruit juice contains 60 mg/100 ml of vitamin C is justified.

Q4.1
Calculate the 95% interval for the mean vitamin C content of the fruit juice.

A4.1
95% confidence interval

$$= \bar{x} \pm t_c \times \frac{s}{\sqrt{n}}$$

$$= 61.5 \pm 2.571 \times \frac{3.391}{\sqrt{6}}$$

$$= [57.94, \ 65.06]$$

(4.5)

4.3.3   *MINITAB commands*

The MINITAB command for performing the tests is shown below.

```
MTB>ttest 60c1

TEST OF MU = 60.00 VS MU N.E.  60.00

        N   MEAN   STDEV  SE MEAN    T    P VALUE
VitC    6   61.50  3.39    1.38    1.08    0.33

MTB>tinterval c1

        N   MEAN   STDEV  SE MEAN   95.0 PERCENT C.I.
VitC    6   61.50  3.39    1.38       (57.94, 65.06)

MTB>ztest 60 3.39c1

TEST OF MU = 60.00 VS MU N.E.  60.00
THE ASSUMED SIGMA = 3.39

        N   MEAN   STDEV  SE MEAN    Z    P VALUE
VitC    6   61.50  3.39    1.38    1.08    0.28

MTB>zinterval 95 3.39c1

THE ASSUMED SIGMA = 3.39

        N   MEAN   STDEV  SE MEAN   95.0 PERCENT C.I.
VitC    6   61.50  3.39    1.38       (58.78, 64.22)
```

4.4   The paired *t*-test

Example 4.3 is used to illustrate hypothesis testing when paired data from underlying normal distributions are available.

Example 4.3

In an experiment to investigate whether smoking affected platelet function, 12 subjects were recruited and the extent to which their blood samples aggregated when exposed to adenosine diphosphate was monitored before and after smoking. Table 4.3 lists the observations. Use a paired *t*-test to evaluate whether smoking did have an effect.

Table 4.3   Effect of smoking on platelet aggregation.

	Subject											
	1	2	3	4	5	6	7	8	9	10	11	12
% Platelet aggregation												
After	70	82	66	69	75	72	77	49	54	66	69	36
Before	60	78	64	68	72	76	74	46	48	60	64	27
Difference	10	4	2	1	3	−4	3	3	6	6	5	9

Solution

Step 1
Set up the null and alternative hypotheses.

$$H_0 : \mu_1 - \mu_2 = \mu_d = 0$$
$$H_1 : \mu_d \qquad > 0 \qquad \text{One-sided test.}$$

where μ_d refers to the mean of the population of differences.

Step 2
Calculate test statistic.

$$t = \frac{\bar{x}_d - 0}{s_d / \sqrt{n}} = \frac{4}{3.69 / \sqrt{12}} = 3.75$$

Step 3
Compare the *t*-statistic against the critical value t_c. $t_c = 2.2$ with 11 degrees of freedom. (Appendix 2 and Fig. 4.6.)

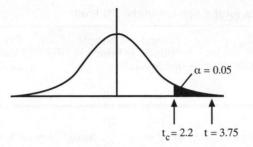

Fig. 4.6 *t*-distribution with 11 degrees of freedom showing the critical value and the observed test statistic.

Step 4
Draw conclusion. The observed *t*-statistic is way beyond 2.2. Therefore H_0 is rejected and H_1 accepted, i.e. smoking increases the aggregability of the platelets. In fact the significance probability is 0.003.

4.5   The sign test

4.5.1   *Background*

The sign test assumes that the variable concerned has a continuous distribution. The underlying principle is very simple. Essentially, if one postulates that the median value is a certain value (*M*) and samples are drawn and measured, then one would expect roughly half of the measurements to be below *M* and the other half above it under the null hypothesis. Values greater than *M* are given the (+) sign and values below the (−) sign; hence the name of the test. The test is essentially a binomial test with the probability *p* of observing a (+) or a (−). The binomial theorem is used to calculate the critical values.

4.5.2   *Mechanics of the test*

Step 1
Set up the null and alternative hypotheses.

H_0: median = K
H_1: median ≠ K or median < K or median > K

Step 2
Calculate the test statistic *s*.
    This is carried out by first assigning a (−) to observed values smaller than K and a (+) to values higher than K. If H_1 is median ≠ K then the test statistic is the smaller of the total number of (+) and the total number of (−). If H_1 is median < K,

Table 4.4   Critical values for the sign test at the 5% level.

Sample size	Critical value (one-sided)	Critical value (two-sided)	Sample size	Critical value (one-sided)	Critical value (two-sided)
5	0	–	18	5	4
6	0	0	19	5	4
7	0	0	20	5	5
8	1	0	21	6	5
9	1	1	22	6	5
10	1	1	23	7	6
11	2	1	24	7	6
12	2	2	25	7	7
13	3	2	26	8	7
14	3	2	27	8	7
15	3	3	28	9	8
16	4	3	29	9	8
17	4	4	30	10	9

then the test statistic is the total number of (+). If H_1 is median > K, then the test statistic is the total number of (–). In other words, for a one-sided sign test, the test statistic is the sum of signs which would be expected to be smaller than M if H_1 were true.

Step 3
Compare the test statistic against the critical value at the significance probability chosen (see Table 4.4). Reject H_0 if the test statistic is equal to or smaller than the critical value.

Step 4
Draw appropriate conclusions.

Note: The sign test may be used to analyse paired data. Differences in the paired observations are calculated first and the sign test is then applied to the single set of differences.

4.5.3   Precautions in the use of the sign test

- The sign test reduces numerical data to either a (+) or a (–) sign. Therefore relatively large differences in the numbers in the (+) and (–) groups are required before H_0 is rejected particularly when the sample size is small.
- When a sample observation coincides with the postulated median (M) simply discard it and carry on with the test using the reduced sample size. If several observations are equal to M then assign half to the (+) group and the other half to the (–) group.

- The test statistic for a one-sided test is the smaller of the number of (+) or (−) signs expected under H_1. For a two-sided test, the test statistic is whichever group ((+) or (−)) gives the smaller value.

4.5.4   Application of the sign test

Example 4.4 shows an application of the sign test.

Example 4.4

In an experiment evaluating the performance of a new anti-acne remedy against a control, subjects with acne were recruited. Their acne was graded using a scale which took account of both number of lesions and the severity of those lesions. Only subjects with the same score on both cheeks were used in the trial. Such subjects were randomly allocated to receive the new remedy or a control product on one cheek and the other product on the other cheek. At the end of one week's treatment the subjects' acne was rescored with the results shown on Table 4.5. Each subject therefore provided a pair of scores.

Table 4.5   Paired acne scores after treatment with a new remedy and a control.

	Acne Score											
New remedy	7	6	6	4	8	5	10	11	11	6	3	6	7
Control product	8	5	6	8	9	6	11	13	13	7	4	9	9
Difference (d)	−1	1	0	−4	−1	−1	−1	−2	−2	−1	−1	−3	−2

Carry out a sign test to test the hypothesis that the new remedy is better than the control product.

Solution

The test is performed on the difference in scores, d.

Step 1

$H_0 : M_d = 0$ i.e. median difference in scores is zero or both treatments are the same.
$H_1 : M_d < 0$ i.e. the new treatment produces a lower median score than the control.

Step 2

Test statistic s = number of positive signs ignoring the tie.
            $s = 1$.

Step 3

Compare the test statistic and the critical value, 2 in this case (see Appendix 9).

Step 4

H_0 is rejected since s is smaller than 2. The new remedy does appear to be better.

Note: Had another two scores provided a (−) sign H_0 could not have been rejected. This shows that relatively large differences in the numbers of (+) and (−) are required before H_0 is rejected. (See section 4.5.3.)

4.6   The Wilcoxon signed rank test: paired data

4.6.1   *Background*

The Wilcoxon signed rank test is essentially a single-sample test for a median value. However, it is most commonly used as a test for matched pairs to investigate whether the median of the population of differences between the paired data is zero. Note that the Mann-Whitney U test and the Wilcoxon sum of ranks test would not be appropriate to analyse paired data as one assumption for both of the latter tests is that the samples are drawn independently.

4.6.2   *Mechanics of the test*

Step 1
Calculate the differences for each pair of data, maintaining the sign.

Step 2
Rank the modulus of the differences (i.e. ignore the sign during the ranking; rank the magnitude). If the difference is zero, ignore and reduce sample size by 1.

Step 3
Sum all the ranks of the differences with negative signs (sum1). Do the same for the differences with positive signs (sum2). The smaller of sum1 and sum2 is the test statistic W.

Step 4
Compare W with the critical value. If W is smaller than the critical value at the significance level chosen, then it is in the critical region and the null hypothesis for no difference in median values is rejected.

Example 4.5

In a study to investigate whether a new sustained release fenfluramine capsule was effective in reducing weight in an obese population, ten individuals from such a population were administered the drug twice daily for one month. Table 4.6 gives data on the patients' weights before and after treatment.

Table 4.6   Patients' weight before and after treatment with fenfluramine.

Patient	Weight before start of therapy (W_A) kg	Weight after end of the month's treatment (W_B) kg
1	92	91.5
2	106	105
3	107	110
4	130	120
5	99	102
6	127	120
7	104	106
8	130	124
9	104	104
10	110	106

Solution

Steps 1 and 2
Table 4.7 shows the weight change for each pair of data and their rank.

Table 4.7   Differences in weight, and corresponding ranks.

Weight change ($W_B - W_A$) kg	Rank
−0.5	1
−1.0	2
3.0	$4\frac{1}{2}$
−10.0	9
3.0	$4\frac{1}{2}$
−7.0	8
2.0	3
−6.0	7
0.0	–
−4.0	6

Step 3
Sum of ranks of differences with negative values

$$= (1 + 2 + 9 + 8 + 7 + 6) = 33$$

Sum of ranks of differences with positive values

$$= (4\frac{1}{2} + 4\frac{1}{2} + 3) = 12$$

The *W* statistic, or the Wilcoxon rank sum statistic, is the smaller sum of the ranks of the positive or negative changes. The ranks are assigned according to the modulus of the changes (i.e. signs ignored as shown above).

The *W* statistic is 12 in this case.

Step 4
The significance probability is therefore greater than 0.10. Since the critical value is 10 (from Appendix 8) at this level of significance, the evidence for a reduction in weight is not very strong.
  Note that the difference equal to zero has been ignored and the sample size reduced by 1. The ties were assigned ranks $4\frac{1}{2}$ each.

Note: While the approach described so far takes account of correlation between the measurements, it does not make allowance for possible *period effects*, that is possible changes in response due solely to the order in which the treatment is given.

Q4.2
Is there a design which can be used to balance out period effects?

A4.2
One approach commonly used to attempt this is by matching pairs of subjects. For example, in a study investigating the possible effect of health education sessions on food intake, pairs of overweight subjects matched on age, extent of obesity, food intake and educational attainment may be recruited and the subjects are then assigned to receive the health educational sessions or an irrelevant control lecture session. The order is chosen randomly for one member of each pair and the reverse order applied to the second member.

Chapter 5
Hypothesis Testing: Two Independent Samples

5.1 Objectives

The two independent samples, or the two-group design, is perhaps the most widely used experimental design. In one subtype of this design, subjects or experimental units are randomly assigned to the two groups and subjected to the different treatments. This approach is commonly used for comparing the effect of different drugs or one drug and a placebo. The responses of the two groups are then compared to test whether the responses are different. In a second subtype, experimental units or subjects are sampled from two distinct populations and are given the same treatment. The responses of the two groups are then compared. This approach is used, for example, for comparing the dissolution rates of two brands of the same tablets or the shelf-life of two different products.

This chapter discusses the choice of hypothesis test to be used for analysing data derived from experiments using such designs. The two-group study design is also used for comparing characteristics of two populations in observational studies. For example, a biologist may wish to compare the wing-spans of two species of a particular insect or an environmentalist may wish to compare the pH of reservoir water in two different countries. Such studies are not called experiments in the statistical sense since no independent variable which affects the response is fixed by the investigators.

5.1.1 Choice of hypothesis test

Figure 5.1 gives a flow diagram of the hypothesis tests to be used in situations commonly encountered with experiments using the two-group design.

Points to note in choosing an appropriate hypothesis test are:

(1) the distribution of the data,
(2) whether the variances of the two populations are equal,
(3) the sample sizes, and
(4) whether the variances are known.

Note: In reading the subsequent material in this chapter, the mechanics of the test will be clearer if the steps involved in carrying out a hypothesis test are borne in mind. These steps are repeated below.

Step 1
Set up the null and alternative hypotheses.

Step 2
Calculate the statistic of interest. In this chapter it is the difference in two population means.

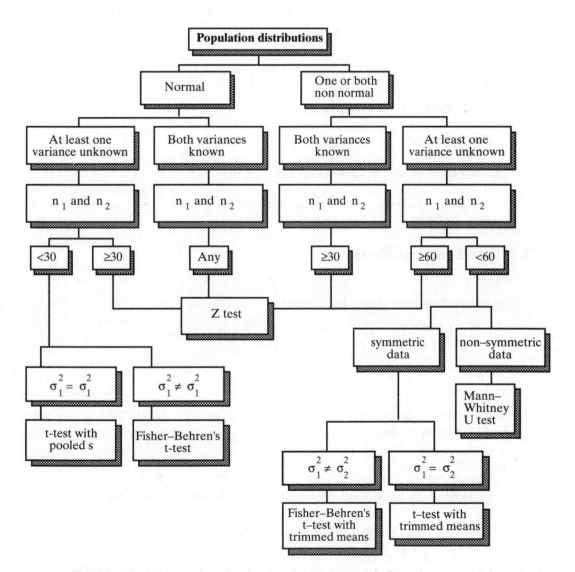

Fig. 5.1   Flow diagram for choosing an appropriate two independent samples hypothesis test.

Step 3
Calculate the *test statistic*, i.e. a statistic whose distribution is known or can be approximated by, for example, the Z-statistic or the t-statistic.

Remember that this is done because one can then work out whether the observations are extreme or consistent with the null hypothesis.

Step 4
Compare the test statistic with the critical value noting that the latter is a value which would be considered extreme enough for rejection of the null hypothesis.

Step 5
Draw conclusions.

5.2   The Z-test – two samples

5.2.1   *Background*

Assumptions about the data:

Unrelated samples of data are drawn from two populations with means, μ_1 and μ_2. Samples drawn are large (≥ 30).

5.2.2   *Mechanics of the test*

Step 1
Set up null and alternative hypotheses.

$$H_0 : \mu_1 = \mu_2 \qquad \text{or} \qquad H_0 : \mu_1 - \mu_2 = 0$$
$$H_1 : \mu_1 \neq \mu_2 \qquad\qquad H_1 : \mu_1 - \mu_2 \neq 0$$

Step 2
Calculate the two means.

If the means of the two populations are the same, then $\mu_1 - \mu_2 = 0$. Therefore, if the sample means ($\bar{x}_1$ and $\bar{x}_2$) are taken, then, on average, one would expect

$$\bar{x}_1 - \bar{x}_2 = 0$$

With sufficiently large samples, the sampling distribution of X is given by

$$\overline{X}_1 \sim N\left(\mu_1, \ \sigma_1^2 / n_1\right)$$
$$\overline{X}_2 \sim N\left(\mu_2, \ \sigma_2^2 / n_2\right)$$

where n_1 and n_2 are the sample sizes.

Therefore, the sampling distribution of $\overline{X}_1 - \overline{X}_2$ is given by

$$\left(\overline{X}_1 - \overline{X}_2\right) \sim N\left(\mu_1 - \mu_2, \ \sigma_1^2/n_1 + \sigma_2^2/n_2\right) \tag{5.1}$$

Step 3
Calculate variance of $(\overline{X}_1 - \overline{X}_2)$, i.e. $\sigma_1^2/n_1 + \sigma_2^2/n_2$

Under the null hypothesis, $\mu_1 - \mu_2 = 0$

$$\therefore \ \left(\overline{X}_1 - \overline{X}_2\right) \sim \left(0, \ \sigma_1^2/n_1 + \sigma_2^2/n_2\right)$$

If σ_1^2 and σ_2^2 are unknown but n_1 and n_2 are greater than 30 then they can be approximated by the sample variances (s_1^2 and s_2^2). For other situations see Fig. 5.1.

Step 4
Standardise.

Standardising gives the test statistic z

$$z = \frac{\left(\overline{x}_1 - \overline{x}_2\right) - \left(\text{hypothesised difference, usually } 0\right)}{\sqrt{\left[\left(\sigma_1^2/n_1\right) + \left(\sigma_2^2/n_2\right)\right]}}$$

$$\frac{\left(\overline{x}_1 - \overline{x}_2\right) - \left(\text{hypothesised difference, usually } 0\right)}{\sqrt{\left[\left(s_1^2/n_1\right) + \left(s_2^2/n_2\right)\right]}} \sim N(0, \ 1)$$

Therefore, the null hypothesis is rejected whenever z is far enough from 0.

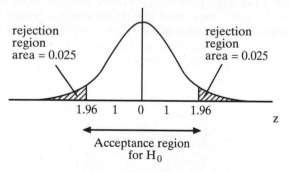

Fig. 5.2   Two-sided Z-test at a significance probability of 0.05.

The critical region, using a two-sided test at the 5% significance level, is given by

$$|z| \geq 1.96$$

Therefore at this significance level H_0 is rejected if the test statistic falls in the shaded region shown in Fig. 5.2.

Step 5
Draw conclusion.

5.2.3 *Other conditions when the Z-test is applicable*

The Z-test is also applicable when:

(1) the populations are not normal but the sample sizes are greater than 30 and the population variances are known and
(2) when the population variances are not known and the populations are not both normal but the sample sizes are both greater than 60 (see Fig. 5.1 diagram).

The Z-statistic in case (2) above is approximated using the sample variances for the difference.

5.3 The two independent samples *t*-test

When the sample sizes are small and at least one of the variances has to be estimated from the samples (i.e. variance unknown) but can be assumed to be equal, the two independent samples *t*-test described in Example 5.1 can be used.

Example 5.1

To determine whether two drugs affected human mental concentration equally, 50 students were given one drug and 50 others the second drug. All the students were then given an examination to measure their mental concentration index. The mean scores for the two groups were $\bar{x}_1 = 65$ and $\bar{x}_2 = 70$, and the respective standard deviations were $s_1 = 15$ and $s_2 = 18$. Is there sufficient evidence to suggest that the two drugs affected mental concentration differently?

Solution

Step 1
$$H_0 : \mu_1 = \mu_2 \qquad \text{or} \qquad H_0 : \mu_1 - \mu_2 = 0$$
$$H_1 : \mu_1 \neq \mu_2 \qquad\qquad\quad H_1 : \mu_1 - \mu_2 \neq 0$$

Step 2
$$\bar{x}_1 - \bar{x}_2 = (65 - 70) = -5$$

Step 3
$$\sigma_1^2/n_1 + \sigma_2^2/n_2 \approx s_1^2/n_1 + s_2^2/n_2$$
$$= 15^2/50 + 18^2/50 = 10.98$$

Step 4

$$z\text{-value} = \frac{-5}{\sqrt{10.98}} = -1.51$$

Step 5
The z-value is within the acceptance region since $z_c = -1.96$ (Appendix 1). Therefore, there is no reason to reject H_0. The evidence would suggest that both drugs have the same effect on mental concentration.

5.4   The two samples *t*-test

5.4.1   *Background*

Assumptions about the data:

The samples are drawn from two populations which are normally distributed with means, μ_1 and μ_2, and having *equal* variance.

Null hypothesis and alternative hypothesis:

$$H_0 : \mu_1 = \mu_2 \qquad \text{or} \qquad H_0 : \mu_1 - \mu_2 = 0$$
$$H_1 : \mu_1 \neq \mu_2 \qquad\qquad H_1 : \mu_1 - \mu_2 \neq 0$$

5.4.2   *Mechanics of the test*

Step 1
Calculate samples means ($\bar{x}_1, \bar{x}_2$) and variances (s_1^2, s_2^2).

Step 2
The assumption in the *t*-test is that the samples come from normal populations with the same variance (s_p^2). Therefore, obtain an estimate using the sample variances.

$$s_p^2 = \frac{(n_1 - 1)s_1^2 + (n_2 - 1)s_2^2}{n_1 + n_2 - 2}$$

Step 3
Calculate the standard error (SE) or the standard deviation of the sampling distribution of ($\bar{x}_1 - \bar{x}_2$)

$$SE = \sqrt{\left[\left(s_p^2/n_1\right) + \left(s_p^2/n_2\right)\right]}$$

Again note that if

$$\overline{X}_1 \sim N\left(\mu_1,\ \sigma_1^2/n_1\right)$$
$$\overline{X}_2 \sim N\left(\mu_2,\ \sigma_2^2/n_2\right)$$

then

$$\left(\overline{X}_1 - \overline{X}_2\right) \sim N\left(\mu_1 - \mu_2,\ \sigma_1^2/n_1 + \sigma_2^2/n_2\right)$$

Step 4
Calculate the *t*-statistic

$$t_\nu = \frac{\left(\overline{x}_1 - \overline{x}_2\right)}{\sqrt{\left[\left(s_p^2/n_1\right) + \left(s_p^2/n_2\right)\right]}} \tag{5.2}$$

where

$$\nu = n_1 + n_2 - 2$$
$$= \text{degrees of freedom.}$$

Again, H_0 is rejected if t is sufficiently removed from zero. The critical values are obtained from statistical tables (see Appendix 2).

For example, at the 5% significance level, with 10 degrees of freedom, the critical value is 2.228 for a two-sided test. At ∞ degrees of freedom the *t*-distribution superimposes on the standard normal distribution, and, hence, the critical value at the same level of significance is 1.96 as expected.

Example 5.2

A report indicated that the elderly are more susceptible to the toxic effects of a particular drug. Pharmacokinetic studies were carried out in a sample of young adults (<30 years of age) and in an elderly sample (>55 years of age) in an attempt to investigate whether there were any differences in the way the two populations handled the drug. One area of particular interest was the kinetics of a potentially toxic metabolite. The 48-hour urinary excretion of the metabolite was

Table 5.1   Metabolite levels in mcg/ml in young and elderly adults.

Pair	Young adults	Elderly
1	8.4	16.3
2	14.5	20.6
3	9.6	14.0
4	8.8	20.1
5	12.0	16.0
6	13.0	14.0
7	10.0	16.5
8	9.8	17.0
9	11.2	16.7
10	11.6	17.8
11	11.7	18.5

as shown in Table 5.1. Was there any evidence that the elderly produced more of the potentially toxic metabolite?

Solution

Table 5.2 Statistics on metabolite levels.

Parameter	Young adults	Elderly
Mean	10.964	17.045
Variance	3.413	4.527
n	11	11
Common variance	$= (10 \times 3.413 + 10 \times 4.527)/20 = 3.97$	
Standard error	$= \sqrt{[(3.97/11) + (3.97/11)]} = 0.850$	
t	$= (10.964 - 17.045)/0.850 = -7.154$	

Significance probability is smaller than 0.001. Therefore, there is strong evidence for higher excretion of the metabolite in the elderly.

5.4.3 Special cases of the t-test

Refer to the flow diagram in Fig. 5.1.

(1)   Unequal unknown variances but distribution normal – the Fisher-Behren's t-test

The t-test assumes normal distributions and equal variances. If the normality assumption holds but at least one of the sample sizes is smaller than 30, and the unknown variances cannot be assumed to be equal, then the t-statistic has to be modified to

$$t' = \frac{(\bar{x}_1 - \bar{x}_2) - (\text{hypothesised difference, usually zero})}{\sqrt{[(s_1^2/n_1) + (s_2^2/n_2)]}}$$

This t-statistic (t') does not follow the t-statistic with $(n_1 + n_2 - 2)$ degrees of freedom as would be the case if the population variances were the same. Instead it follows a distribution called the *Fisher-Behren's distribution* which is approximated by the usual t-distribution with ν degrees of freedom such that

$$\nu = \frac{\left(s_1^2/n_1 + s_2^2/n_2\right)^2}{\left[\dfrac{\left(s_1^2/n_1\right)^2}{n_1 - 1} + \dfrac{\left(s_2^2/n_2\right)^2}{n_2 - 1}\right]} \tag{5.3}$$

v calculated using this formula is not usually an integer and is rounded to the nearest integer.

(2) The unknown population variances *can* be assumed equal but the populations are not normal though symmetric; $30 < n_1$ and $n_2 < 50$

The statistician C.P. Winsor made the now validated observation that all frequency distributions are normal in the middle. This has led others to propose the use of trimmed data, i.e. data from which outliers have been removed. This approach has been shown to be valid provided the distribution is symmetric.

The use of this approach for carrying out a hypothesis test about the means of two populations is as follows.

Step 1
Delete 10% of the data at each end of each sample data to reduce the sample sizes n_1 and n_2 to m_1 and m_2.

Step 2
Calculate the means of the trimmed data to give $\bar{x}_{1t}$ and $\bar{x}_{2t}$.

Step 3
Replace the data removed from each data set by an equal number of new data, each having the value of the last data point at the trimmed end. The new data sets are called *Winsorised data sets*. This is shown in Table 5.3.

Table 5.3 The creation of Winsorised data sets.

Original sample:	**39 44 46**│	47, 47, 47, 48, 48, 48, 48, 49, 49, 50, 50, 50, 50, 51, 51, 51, 51, 53, 53, 53, 55, 55, 55, 57, │**60 68 76**
Trimmed sample:	────────────│	47, 47, 47, 48, 48, 48, 48, 49, 49, 50, 50, 50, 50, 51, 51, 51, 51, 53, 53, 53, 55, 55, 55, 57, │────────
Winsorised sample:	**47 47 47**│	47, 47, 48, 48, 48, 48, 49, 49, 50, 50, 50, 50, 51, 51, 51, 51, 53, 53, 53, 55, 55, 55, 57, │**57 57 57**

Step 4
Calculate the variance of the Winsorised sets to give s^2_{1w} and s^2_{2w}.

Step 5
Calculate the pooled estimate of the common variance of the two populations using the Winsorised data.

$$s^2 = \frac{(n_1 - 1)s_{1w}^2 + (n_2 - 1)s_{2w}^2}{m_1 + m_2 - 2}$$
(5.4)

Step 6
Calculate the test statistic

$$t = \frac{(\bar{x}_{1t} - \bar{x}_{2t}) - (\text{hypothesised value usually zero})}{\sqrt{[(s^2/m_1) + (s^2/m_2)]}}$$
(5.5)

Step 7
Compare the test statistic with the appropriate critical value using the t-distribution with $(m_1 + m_2 - 2)$ degrees of freedom.

Step 8
Draw conclusion.

(3)   Unknown population variances which *cannot* be assumed to be equal but the populations are not normal though symmetric; $30 < n_1$ and $n_2 < 60$

The same procedure as described under (2) is appropriate except that the Fisher-Behren statistic t' is used.

$$t' = \frac{(\bar{x}_{1t} - \bar{x}_{2t}) - (\text{hypothesised value usually zero})}{\sqrt{(s_{\bar{x}_{1t}}^2 + s_{\bar{x}_{2t}}^2)}}$$

where

$$s_{1t}^2 = \frac{s_{1w}^2}{m_1} \times \frac{(n_1 - 1)}{(m_1 - 1)} \qquad \text{and} \qquad s_{2t}^2 = \frac{s_{2w}^2}{m_2} \times \frac{(n_2 - 1)}{(m_2 - 1)}$$

The t' statistic approximates the usual t-distribution with ν degrees of freedom where

$$\nu = \frac{\left(s_{\bar{x}_{1t}}^2 + s_{\bar{x}_{2t}}^2\right)^2}{\left(\dfrac{s_{\bar{x}_{1t}}^2}{m_1 - 1} + \dfrac{s_{\bar{x}_{2t}}^2}{m_2 - 2}\right)}$$

(4)   Unknown population variances, non-symmetrical distributions and n_1 or $n_2 < 60$

5.5   The Mann-Whitney U-test

5.5.1   Background

The t-test assumes that the distributions studied are normal and have equal variances. When there are doubts about these assumptions, a non-parametric test is required and the Mann-Whitney test is one of the most powerful available.

If two independent samples consisting of n_1 and n_2 observations are collected from populations 1 and 2 and the observations are pooled $(n_1 + n_2)$ and ranked, then comparison of the ranks would enable one to make inferences about whether the two populations show differences in location or average value. If the two populations show no difference in means, then the number of times observations from population 1 are ranked higher than those from population 2 would be expected to be equal to the number of times the reverse situation occurs. This forms the basis of the Mann-Whitney U-test.

5.5.2   Mechanics of the test

Step 1
Compare each value from population 1 with every value from population 2 and count the total number of times (n_1) values from population 1 exceed values from population 2. There are therefore $n_1 n_2$ comparisons to be made. This is made manageable by a stem plot (see Example 5.3).

Step 2
Subtract n_1 from $n_1 n_2$ to give n_2, the number of times population 2 values exceed population 1 values.

The Mann-Whitney statistic, U, is the smaller of n_1 and n_2.

Step 3
Compare U with the critical value (Appendix 7). The question being asked is what is the probability of seeing a U value as small as that obtained in the comparison. The critical region therefore covers values *smaller* than the critical value.

Example 5.3

A number of marathon runners collapse during or at the finish of competitive racing. It is postulated that these runners are able to run until they collapse because they secrete increased amounts of endogenous opioids to counteract pain which would otherwise stop the running well before the collapse stage. To test this hypothesis, the β endorphin levels are measured in a group of runners immediately after they collapse. The β endorphin levels of the same number of runners who did not show signs of extreme exhaustion at the end of the race were also measured. The data were as shown in Table 5.4.

Table 5.4 β endorphin levels in marathon runners.

Subject	β endorphin plasma levels (pmol/l)	
	Control runners	Collapsed runners
1	14	109
2	20	70
3	50	47
4	17	36
5	45	130
6	35	108
7	37	29
8	16	55
9	26	42
10	24	118

Solution

Step 1
Stem plot

Collapsed runners		Control runners	Number of values in collapsed runners below those in control runners
	1	5 8 9	0, 0, 0
9	2	0 4 6	0, 0, 0
6	3	5 7	1, 2
7 2	4	5	3
5	5	0	4
	6		
0	7		For those not familiar with stem plots:
	8		note the first line under control
	9		runners reproduces the values 15, 18
8	10		and 19
8 0	11		
	12		
	13		
0	14		

Step 2
U-statistic = 1 + 2 + 3 + 4 = 10

It is quite clear that this is the *U*-statistic since there are 10 × 10 comparisons and in only 10 of these does the β endorphin level in the collapsed runner fall below that of the control runner. In the other 90 cases the reverse position is true.

An alternative scheme ranks the data as shown below:

Control runners	15	18	19	20	24	26	35	37	45	50
Collapsed runners							29	36	42	47
No. of values in collapsed runners below those of controls	0	0	0	0	0	0	1	2	3	4

Values above 50 are all from collapsed runners and can be ignored. Therefore the *U*-statistic equals 10 as before.

Step 3
The critical value (from Neave, 1979) is 16 at a significance probability of 0.01. Hence H_0 of the same β endorphin level in the two populations of runners is rejected. Indeed it appears that β endorphin helps endurance (see Dale *et al.*, 1987).

5.6   The Wilcoxon sum of ranks test

5.6.1   Background

This test is essentially the same as the Mann-Whitney rank sum test. The assumption is again that the samples are drawn independently. If the data are paired, then these two tests are not appropriate and the Wilcoxon *signed* rank test should be used instead. However, because the Wilcoxon *sum* of ranks test is still commonly used, an example is given in Example 5.4.

5.6.2   Mechanics of the test

Step 1
Rank all values from both samples into a single ascending series. The smallest value is ranked 1.

Step 2
Sum the ranks for the two samples to give R_A and R_B and use the smaller one as the test statistic R.

Step 3
Compare the test statistic against the critical value obtained from suitable tables. If the observed value of R is smaller than the critical value, then H_0: the samples are drawn from the same population, is rejected.

The Wilcoxon sum of ranks test statistic (R) can be converted to the Mann-Whitney rank sum statistic (U) by the formula

$$U_B = R_B - \frac{1}{2} n_B (n_B + 1) \tag{5.6}$$

or

$$U_A = R_A - \frac{1}{2} n_A (n_A + 1) \tag{5.7}$$

where n_A and n_B are the sample sizes. A Mann-Whitney table of critical values can then be used (Appendix 7).

Example 5.4

To investigate whether the smoking habits of mothers affected the weight of newborns, the weight of 20 baby boys from mothers of the same socio-economic group and general health were recorded, see Table 5.5. Is there evidence that smoking affects birth weight?

Table 5.5   Weight of baby boys born to smoking and non-smoking mothers in kg.

Non-smoking mothers Sample A	Smoking mothers Sample B
3.65	3.35
3.45	2.15
4.50	2.70
4.10	2.90
3.50	3.25
3.10	3.75
2.90	3.00
3.20	3.35
3.30	3.10
4.00	2.30

Solution

Step 1

2.15	2.30	2.70	2.90	2.90	3.00	3.10	3.10	3.20	3.25
1	2	3	$4\frac{1}{2}$	$4\frac{1}{2}$	6	$7\frac{1}{2}$	$7\frac{1}{2}$	9	10
B	B	B	B	A	B	B	A	A	B

3.30	3.35	3.35	3.45	3.50	3.65	3.75	4.00	4.10	4.50
11	$12\frac{1}{2}$	$12\frac{1}{2}$	14	15	16	17	18	19	20
A	B	B	A	A	A	B	A	A	A

Step 2

Sum of ranks for sample A = 134 = R_A

Sum of ranks for sample B = 76 = R_B

Converting to Mann-Whitney statistic

$$U_B = R_B - \frac{1}{2} n_B (n_B + 1) = 21 \tag{5.8}$$

Step 3
Critical value at a significance probability of 0.05 is 23 (two-sided test appendix 7).
Since U_B is smaller than the critical value, H_0 is rejected.
The evidence is that smoking does affect the babies' weights.

Note that if the weights can be assumed to follow the normal distributions, then the *t*-test would be better because of its higher power.

5.6.3   Points to watch

- In observational studies, the samples must be chosen at random using an appropriate sampling procedure. In experimental studies using the two-group design, subjects must be assigned randomly to the two groups, again using an established procedure for such assignments (see Appendix 10). If necessary pretest the equivalence of the two groups even after random assignment and repeat the procedure if required.
- Non-random subject loss during the study may invalidate a study. Dropout and withdrawal from treatment are usually non-random. A post test assessment of equivalence in factors which may affect the response is worthwhile. If differences are observed, these ought to be highlighted in the report.
- In many studies several groups are studied simultaneously and it is tempting to break those groups into pairs which are then analysed by the methods described in this chapter. This temptation must be resisted as the α value for the whole study would be inflated relative to the single comparison study; that is there is an increased risk of erroneously concluding that a difference exists between the populations studied. Analysis of variance followed by a multiple comparison method is usually the appropriate approach to analysing such data (see Chapter 7).

5.6.4   Hypothesis test for differences between population proportions

The same tests as those used for population means can be used except that the standard error terms are different. The appropriate tests for various situations are summarised below. The following symbols are used:

π_1 and π_2	Population proportions with attribute of interest.
p_1 and p_2	The sample proportions with attribute of interest.
n_1 and n_2	The sample sizes.
s	Sample standard deviation.

For large samples $n_1 p_1$ and $n_2 p_2 \geq 5$

$n_1(1 - p_1)$ and $n_2(1 - p_2) \geq 5$ the following apply.

Test statistic

$$\frac{(p_1 - p_2) - (\text{Hypothesised value usually zero})}{\sqrt{\left[\dfrac{p(1-p)}{n_1} + \dfrac{p(1-p)}{n_2}\right]}} \qquad (5.9)$$

where

$$p = \frac{n_1 p_1 + n_2 p_2}{n_1 + n_2}$$

Critical value

$Z_{1-\alpha/2}$ for a two-sided test.
$Z_{1-\alpha}$ for an upper-tailed one-sided test.
$-Z_{1-\alpha}$ for a lower-tailed one-sided test.

100(1 – α)% confidence interval

$$(p_1 + p_2) \pm z_{1-\alpha/2} \sqrt{\left[\frac{p_1(1-p_1)}{n_1} + \frac{p_2(1-p_2)}{n_2}\right]} \qquad (5.10)$$

Chapter 6
Correlation and Regression

6.1 Objectives

The Pearson moment correlation coefficient is defined and cautions in its use highlighted. Simple linear regression analysis is described along with the assumptions made in its development. The use of the computer programs SAS and MINITAB in simple linear regression is illustrated and details of the calculations of the statistics shown in the computer outputs are explained. Consideration of the calculations may be delayed until a second read of this chapter. Methods for arriving at estimates of the parameters concerned and for making appropriate inferences using simple regression analysis are discussed. In particular after reading this chapter, the reader should be able to:

(1) Test for linear association between two variables.
(2) Calculate confidence intervals for the slope β and intercept α.
(3) Calculate confidence and prediction intervals for mean and individual y values.
(4) Make interpolations and extrapolations and know of the dangers associated with the latter.
(5) Test for equality or otherwise of two slopes β_1 and β_2.
(6) Test for an outlier with paired data.
(7) Understand the basis of multiple linear regression.
(8) Perform non-linear regression analyses using computer packages.

The choice of appropriate measure of association and regression model is shown in Figs 6.1 and 6.2 respectively.

Notation

For notation used in this chapter see below and later in Table 6.2.

α	y intercept of population regression line $y = \alpha + \beta x$.
β	Slope of population regression line.
$\bar{y}$	Mean of y values.
$\bar{x}$	Mean of x values.
Σ	Summation symbol.
r	Correlation coefficient.

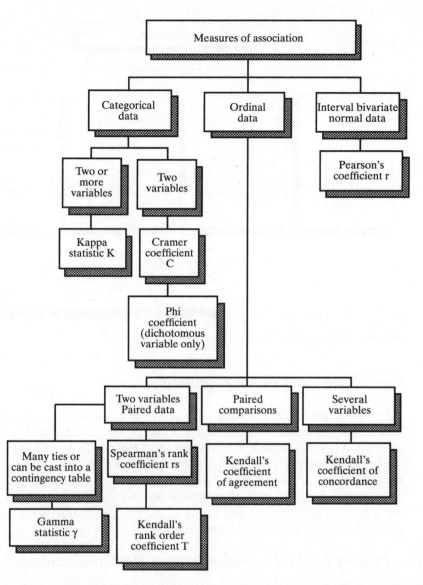

Fig. 6.1 Flow of diagram for choosing an appropriate measure of association between variables.

r^2	Coefficient of determination.
σ^2	Variance of mean y values.
$s_{\hat{y}}$	Standard error of mean value y corresponding to point (x, y).
s_{y_i}	Standard error of single y value corresponding to point (x_i, y_i).
R_i	Residual of point (x_i, y_i) from fitted line.

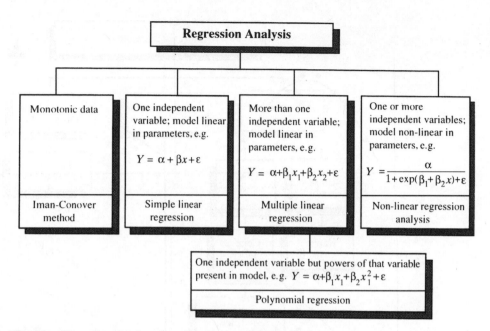

Fig. 6.2   Flow diagram for choosing a regression method.

6.2   Correlation and linear regression

Very often, one wishes to measure the degree of association between two variables (x and y). For example, is the score achieved by an individual in mathematics associated with the score achieved in physics? Is the height of a son associated with the height of his father? To answer such questions, *correlation analysis* is used. The most common measure of *linear* association between two variables is the *Pearson moment correlation coefficient* or *correlation coefficient* for short. The symbol used for a population is rho (ρ) and for a sample (r). The correlation coefficient (r) is calculated using the formula shown in Table 6.3.

6.2.1   *Properties of the correlation coefficient and cautions*

(1)   Interchanging variables (x and y) does not change its value.

(2)   Changing the unit of measurement does not affect its value.

(3)   The range of values taken by r is -1 to 1; an r value of -1 or 1 indicates a perfect linear relationship.

(4)   A negative r value indicates that as one of the variables decreases the other increases while a positive r value indicates that both variables move together in the same direction.

(5)   A zero regression coefficient indicates absence of a linear relationship between two variables. However, there may well be a strong non-linear association (e.g. parabolic) between the two variables (Fig. 6.3(a)).

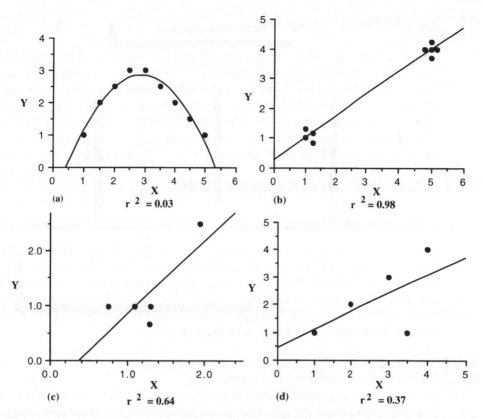

Fig. 6.3 Potential spurious correlations when applying correlation analysis to inappropriate data. (a) Correlated but not linear data; (b) clustered data; (c) one outlier gives spurious correlation and (d) one outlier reduces coefficient markedly.

(6) The strength of linear association between two variables with a correlation coefficient of –0.8 is as strong as one with a correlation of +0.8.

(7) The existence of a correlation between two variables does not mean that one variable causes the other.

(8) Combining data which could be subdivided into distinct sets on the basis of some other variable may lead to spurious correlations between two variables (Fig. 6.3(b)).

(9) An extreme score may give evidence for a correlation when none exists (Fig. 6.3(c)). Alternatively, an extreme score may suggest absence of a correlation between two variables although there is a strong correlation for the other scores (Fig. 6.3(d)).

(10) Restricting the range of the two variables will reduce the correlation coefficient obtained.

(11) Data should be plotted as part of correlation analysis.

6.3   Simple linear regression

Simple linear regression is essentially fitting a straight line through paired data (e.g. two test scores for the same individual) using dependent samples (e.g. scores in test 1 and scores in test 2 with the same individuals). In regression one therefore attempts to explain the variation in one variable (e.g. score in test 2) using another variable (e.g. score in test 1). In simple linear regression, the straight line equation which is obtained may then be used to predict the value taken by the second variable (score in test 2) when given the value of the first variable (score in test 1).

6.3.1   The simple linear regression model

$$y = \alpha + \beta x + \varepsilon$$

The simple linear regression model assumes that there is a straight line with slope β and intercept α to define the population data. When x is fixed the y value observed will be given by the equation plus a random error term ε. This error is normally distributed with mean 0 and variance σ^2. In other words, for any given x_i value the observed y value will have a normal distribution mean value of $(\alpha + \beta x_i)$ and a variance of σ^2 as illustrated in Fig. 6.4.

6.3.2   Fitting a straight line through paired data

Given a set of sample paired data (e.g. scores in two tests by the same individuals) how does one obtain the equation of the straight line? Any straight line may be represented by an equation of the form:

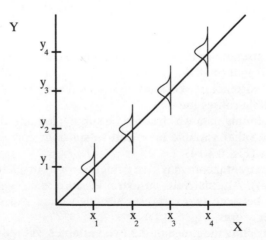

Fig. 6.4   Illustration of the assumption that with linear regression the errors associated with the y terms are identically distributed normal variates.

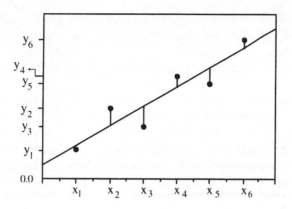

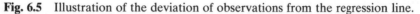

Fig. 6.5 Illustration of the deviation of observations from the regression line.

$$y = a + bx \qquad \text{or} \qquad y = \alpha + \beta x$$
$$\text{for a sample} \qquad \qquad \text{for a population} \tag{6.1}$$

The most common approach to obtaining this equation for a set of paired data is the *method of least squares*. Essentially, this method involves obtaining a and b values such that the sum of squared deviations (SSE) of the observed y values from the line is a minimum (Fig. 6.5).

The square deviations are the square of the individual distances from the points to the line.

The method of calculation for determining a and b are set out later in Table 6.3.

6.3.3 Coefficient of determination

The coefficient of determination, r^2, is simply the square of the Pearson product moment correlation coefficient, r. While r gives us an indication of the strength of linear association between two variables (x and y), r^2 goes further and gives us a precise interpretation of the association in terms of variances. The coefficient of determination (r^2) is the fraction of the variation in y explained by the fitted equation. For example, if r is 0.3, the coefficient of determination is 0.09. Therefore, only 9% (0.09) of the changes in y are associated with changes in x, in this instance. The linear relationship between x and y is therefore very weak.

6.3.4 Possible objectives in a simple linear regression analysis

Various inferences and estimates may be made from the regression lines:

(1) Estimate σ^2, the population variance for the y values.
(2) Estimate the variability associated with the estimated slope (b) and intercept (a).
(3) Test whether there is any association between the two variables x and y.

(4) Estimate the variability associated with a given y value.
(5) Make predictions about the y value for a given x value within the range studied.
(6) Make predictions about the mean y value given an x value.

In order to make those inferences and estimates, the y values are assumed to be normally distributed with equal variance (Fig. 6.4). The y values should be independent and in the underlying population the x and y values should be linearly related. Before considering the formulae for making those inferences and estimates let us first consider an example of a linear regression with computer outputs.

Example 6.1

In an experiment investigating the breakdown of aspirin in a pharmaceutical product stored at 25°C, the data held in file CUL32.dat were obtained (see Table 6.1).

Table 6.1   File CUL32.dat. Data on aspirin decomposition.

Observation	Time	Aspirin remaining
1	18	603.61
2	35	601.12
3	51	597.95
4	68	594.32
5	85	591.38
6	101	587.30
7	118	581.85
8	136	580.04
9	166	578.45
10	197	570.52
11	229	561.45
12	260	557.37
13	292	549.21
14	326	546.03
15	355	541.04

Solution

A linear regression analysis was carried out using SAS software as follows.

SAS commands

	Objective
`data test1;`	
`infile 'a:cul32.dat';`	Location of file.
`input time aspirin;`	Read in time and aspirin data.
`proc print;`	Printing of values read.
`proc reg;`	Command to initiate regression analysis.
`model aspirin = time / p r cli clm;`	Model to be used.
`run;`	

The time and aspirin data were in file CUL32.dat in drive a:. Below is a specimen output.

SAS output

Model: MODEL1
Dependent Variable: ASPIRIN

Analysis of Variance

Source	DF	Sum of Squares	Mean Square	F Value	Prob > F
Model	1	6025.41662	6025.41662	2384.279	0.0001
Error	13	32.85288	2.52714		
C Total	14	6058.26949			

Root MSE	1.58970	R-square	0.9946
Dep Mean	576.10933	Adj R-sq	0.9942
C.V.	0.27594		

Parameter Estimates

Variable	DF	Parameter Estimate	Standard Error	T for H0: Parameter = 0	Prob > T
INTERCEP	1	607.001080	0.75413734	804.895	0.0001
TIME	1	−0.190142	0.00389403	−48.829	0.0001

Obs	Dep Var ASPIRIN	Predict Value	Std Err Predict	Lower95% Mean	Upper95% Mean	Lower95% Predict	Upper95% Predict
1	603.6	603.6	0.696	602.1	605.1	599.8	607.3
2	601.1	600.3	0.644	599.0	601.7	596.6	604.1
3	598.0	597.3	0.597	596.0	598.6	593.6	601.0
4	594.3	594.1	0.551	592.9	595.3	590.4	597.7
5	591.4	590.8	0.509	589.7	591.9	587.2	594.4
6	587.3	587.8	0.475	586.8	588.8	584.2	591.4
7	581.8	584.6	0.445	583.6	585.5	581.0	588.1
8	580.0	581.1	0.423	580.2	582.1	577.6	584.7
9	578.5	575.4	0.411	574.6	576.3	571.9	579.0
10	570.5	569.5	0.432	568.6	570.5	566.0	573.1
11	561.5	563.5	0.485	562.4	564.5	559.9	567.0
12	557.4	557.6	0.559	556.4	558.8	553.9	561.2
13	549.2	551.5	0.650	550.1	552.9	547.8	555.2
14	546.0	545.0	0.758	543.4	546.7	541.2	548.8
15	541.0	539.5	0.855	537.7	541.3	535.6	543.4

The same regression analysis was carried out with the program MINITAB.

MINITAB commands

	Objective
MTB>regress c2 1 c1;	Command to regress data in column 2 on C1.
SUBC>predict 35;	Command to predict aspirin remaining when time = 35.
SUBC>predict 250;	Command to predict aspirin remaining when time = 250.
SUBC>predict 710.	Command to predict aspirin remaining when time = 710.

MINITAB output

```
The regression equation is
aspmg = 607 - 0.190 timemin
```

Predictor	Coef	Stdev	t-ratio	p
Constant	607.001	0.754	804.89	0.000
timemin	-0.190142	0.003894	-48.83	0.000

```
s = 1.590        R-sq = 99.5%        R-sq(adj) = 99.4%
```

Analysis of Variance

SOURCE	DF	SS	MS	F	p
Regression	1	6025.4	6025.4	2384.27	0.000
Error	13	32.9	2.5		
Total	14	6058.3			

Obs.	timemin	aspmg	Fit	Stdev.Fit	Residual	St.Resid
1	18	603.610	603.578	0.696	0.031	0.02
2	35	601.120	600.346	0.644	0.774	0.53
3	51	597.950	597.304	0.597	0.646	0.44
4	68	594.320	594.071	0.551	0.249	0.17
5	85	591.380	590.839	0.509	0.541	0.36
.						
.						
.						
14	326	546.030	545.015	0.758	1.015	0.73
15	355	541.040	539.501	0.855	1.539	1.15

Fit	Stdev.Fit	95% C.I.	95% P.I.	
600.346	0.644	(598.954,601.738)	(596.640,604.053)	
559.466	0.534	(558.313,560.619)	(555.842,563.089)	
472.000	2.171	(467.308,476.692)	(466.185,477.815)	XX

```
X denotes a row with X values away from the center
XX denotes a row with very extreme X values
```

Interpreting the outputs for model y = a + bx

Table 6.2 lists the terms used by the MINITAB and SAS software packages.

Table 6.2 Definition of terms output by MINITAB and SAS.

Term		Computer package abbreviation	
		MINITAB	SAS
df	Degrees of freedom	df	df
SSReg	Regression sum of squares	Regression SS	Model sum of squares
SSE	Error sum of squares	Error SS	Error sum of squares
SSTo	Total sum of squares	Total SS	C Total sum of squares
MSReg	Mean square regression	Regression MS	Model mean square
MSE	Mean square error	Error MS	Error mean square
C.V.%	Coefficient of variation %		C.V
F	F-value = MSR/MSE	F	F value
a	Parameter estimate for y intercept	Constant coefficient	Intercept parameter estimate
b	Parameter estimate for slope	'X' coefficient	'X' parameter estimate
s_a	Standard error for estimate of intercept α	Constant stdev.	Intercept standard error
s_b	Standard error for estimate of slope	'X' stdev.	'X' standard error
SD	Standard deviation of a predicted *mean* or fitted y value	Stdev.Fit	Std Err predict
s	Standard deviation of an *individual* y value	s	Root MSE
$\hat{y}$	Predicted mean y value at given x value	Fit	Predict value
95% C.I.	Lower and upper 95% confidence values for mean y value at given x value	95% C.I	Lower and upper 95% mean
95% P.I.	Lower and upper prediction values for a single y value	95% P.I	Lower and upper 95% predict
t ratio	t value observed for test of hypothesis H_0: intercept $0 = 0$	Constant t ratio	Intercep T for H_0: Parameter = 0
	t value observed for test of hypothesis H_0: slope $\beta = 0$	'X' t ratio	'X' T for H_0: Parameter = 0
p	Probability of obtaining a t-value greater than the observed t-ratio	p	Prob > |T|

How the values are calculated

Table 6.3 shows how the different statistics are calculated.

Table 6.3

$$s_x = \sum(x_i - \bar{x})/(n-1)$$

$$s_y = \sum(y_i - \bar{y})/(n-1)$$

$$r = \frac{\sum(x_i - \bar{x})(y_i - \bar{y})}{\sqrt{\left[(x_i - \bar{x})^2(y_i - \bar{y})^2\right]}}$$

$$\mathrm{COV}(x, y) = \frac{\sum(x_i - \bar{x})(y_i - \bar{y})}{(n-1)}$$

$$b = r_{s_y/s_x} = \frac{\sum(x_i - \bar{x})(y_i - \bar{y})}{\sum(x_i - \bar{x})^2}$$

$$a = \bar{y} - b\bar{x}$$

$$\mathrm{SSTo} = \sum(y_i - \bar{y})^2$$

$$\mathrm{SSReg} = \sum(\hat{y}_i - \bar{y})^2$$

$$\mathrm{SSE} = \sum(y_i - \hat{y}_i)^2$$

$$\mathrm{SSTo} = \mathrm{SSReg} + \mathrm{SSE}$$

$$\mathrm{MSReg} = \mathrm{SSReg}/1 = (1 - r^2)/(n-2)$$

$$\mathrm{MSE} = \mathrm{SSE}/(n-2)$$

$$\frac{\mathrm{SSReg}}{\mathrm{SSTo}} + \frac{\mathrm{SSE}}{\mathrm{SSTo}} = 1$$

$$F = \mathrm{MSReg}/\mathrm{MSE} = \frac{(n-2)r^2}{(l - r^2)}$$

$$s_b = \sqrt{s^2/\sum(x_i - \bar{x})^2}$$

$$s_{\hat{y}} = \sqrt{\mathrm{MSE}\left[1/n + \frac{(x_i - \bar{x})^2}{\sum(x_i - \bar{x})^2}\right]}$$

$$s_{y_i} = \sqrt{s_{\hat{y}}^2 + \mathrm{MSE}}$$

$$\mathrm{C.V\%} = \left[\sqrt{\mathrm{MSE}}/\mathrm{mean}\right] \times 100$$

Making inferences and estimates: model $y = \alpha + \beta x$

Simple linear regression analysis produces estimates *a* for parameter α and *b* for parameter β. We also obtain the correlation coefficient *r* for the two variables *x* and *y*. How good are those estimates and how can one test whether there is indeed a linear relationship between the two variables? The following highlights methods for carrying out such estimates and hypothesis tests.

(a) Testing for linear association

Step 1

The appropriate null hypothesis is.

$H_0: \beta = 0$ i.e. no linear association between *x* and *y*.

Step 2

The alternative hypothesis is

$H_1: \beta \neq 0$ i.e. there is a linear association between the two variables.

Step 3
The test statistic is the *F*-value

$$F = \text{MSReg}/\text{MSE} = \frac{(n-2)r^2}{1-r^2} \qquad (6.2)$$

Step 4
The critical *F*-value is read from tables with 1 and $(n-2)$ degrees of freedom. The null hypothesis is rejected if the test statistic is greater than *F* critical. In the present example (see MINITAB output above), with $n = 15$ the $F_{1,13}$ value at the $\alpha = 0.05$ level is 4.67 (see Appendix 3). Since the observed *F*-value is 2384.27, there is very strong evidence of linear association between aspirin and time.

(b) Calculating a confidence interval for b, the estimate of the true slope β

The confidence interval for *b* is given by $b \pm t \times$ [standard error of the estimate for β] $= b \pm t s_b$. The appropriate *t* value is based on $(n-2)$ degrees of freedom. In the aspirin example (see SAS or MINITAB output above)

> $b = -0.190142$
> $t_{\alpha=0.05, 13df} = 2.160$ from Appendix 2.
> $s_b = 0.00389403$ from SAS output or 0.003894 from MINITAB output

Therefore the 95% confidence interval $= -0.190142 \pm (2.160) \times 0.003894$
$$= [-0.199, -0.182].$$

(c) Calculating confidence interval for a, the estimate of the intercept α

The confidence interval for *a* is given by $a \pm t \times$ [standard error of the estimate for α]. So in our aspirin example,

> $t_{\alpha=0.05, 13df} = 607.001 \pm 2.160 \times 0.754$ from MINITAB output
>
> $= [605.372, 608.630].$

(d) Confidence interval (CI) for the estimate of mean y value given an x value x_i

Suppose that the mean value is $\hat{y}_i = a + bx_i$. Point $(x_i, \hat{y}_i)$ is on regression line confidence interval for $y_i = \hat{y}_i \pm t \times$ [standard error] $= \hat{y}_i \pm t_{n-2} \times s_{\hat{y}_i}$. Thus in our example, for aspirin, the amount of aspirin left at time 35 (using MINITAB output)

> $= 600.346 \pm 2.160 \times 0.644$
>
> $= [598.954, 601.738].$

These values are the same as shown in the MINITAB output using the predict subcommand predict 39; (see MINITAB commands above for the example).

(e) Prediction value (PI) for a single y value corresponding to a given x value x_i

The value of *y* predicted using the regression line is given by $y_i = a + bx_i$. The prediction interval is calculated using the formula

$$PI = y_i \pm t \times [\text{standard error for estimate}]$$

$$= [a + bx_i] \pm t_{n-2} \times \sqrt{(MSE + s_{\hat{y}}^2)} \tag{6.3}$$

Thus in our aspirin example (see MINITAB and SAS outputs), our 95% prediction interval when $x_i = 35$ is given by

$$600.346 \pm 2.160 \times \sqrt{(2.52714 + 0.644^2)}$$

$$= [596.641, \ 604.051]$$

the same prediction interval as shown in the last section of the MINITAB output.

(f)   Interpolation or estimating y value corresponding to x_i within the x range studied

If the mean y value is required then the estimate is $\hat{y}_i = a + bx_i$. Confidence intervals are calculated as under (d) and prediction intervals as under (e) above.

(g)   Extrapolation or estimating y value corresponding to x_i outside the x range studied

Extrapolation always carries a significant risk of drawing erroneous conclusions. Therefore in practice great care is required when doing so. However, in many instances estimates are made despite the known risks. One example is that on aspirin. One may wish to find out how much is left after 710 minutes (see MINITAB commands). The prediction shows that 472 mg are expected to be left with the confidence and prediction intervals shown in the MINITAB output. Note that MINITAB prints out a warning about the x value being very extreme.

(h)   Comparing two slopes

Suppose that two regression lines $y = a_1 + b_1 x$ and $y = a_2 + b_2 x$ are obtained as estimates for hypothesised population regression lines $y = \alpha_1 + \beta_1 x$ and $y = \alpha_1 + \beta_2 x$. To test for whether β_1 and β_2 are from the same population (i.e. lines are parallel), the following hypothesis test is carried out.

Step 1
Set up null hypothesis.

$$H_0 : \beta_1 = \beta_2 \qquad \text{or equivalently} \qquad (\beta_1 - \beta_2) = 0$$

Step 2
Set up alternative hypothesis.

$$H_1 : (\beta_1 - \beta_2) \neq 0$$

Step 3
Calculate test statistic.

$$z = \frac{(b_1 - b_2) - 0}{\sqrt{(s_{b_1}^2 + s_{b_2}^2)}} \tag{6.4}$$

This statistic can be assumed to be approximately normally distributed with mean zero and variance 1.

Step 4
Compare against critical value (Appendix 1). If the test statistic, ignoring the sign, is greater than 1.96 then H_0 can be rejected at $\alpha = 0.05$ level.

(i) Testing for an outlier

The residual R_i for point y_i when $x = x_i$ is given by

$$R_i = y_i - (a + bx_i)$$

The expected value (mean) of R_i is zero and its variance is given by

$$V(R_i) = \left(1 - \frac{1}{n} - \frac{(x_i - \bar{x})^2}{\sum (x - \bar{x})^2} \right) r^2$$

$$\cong \left(1 - \frac{1}{n} - \frac{(x_i - \bar{x})^2}{\sum (x - \bar{x})^2} \right) s^2 \tag{6.5}$$

If the model is correct then

$$r_i / \sqrt{V(R_i)} \approx \mathrm{N}(0,\ 1) \tag{6.6}$$

Therefore at the 5% significance level, point y_i is taken to be an outlier if $r_i/\sqrt{V(R_i)}$ is greater than 1.96 or smaller than -1.96.

6.4 Spearman's rank correlation coefficient

As already discussed, the Pearson's correlation coefficient is based on some rather restrictive assumptions about the two variables being considered. Spearman's rank correlation coefficient (r_s) overcomes most of the restrictions. With this approach one simply examines whether there is a tendency for the two variables to increase or decrease together (positive correlation) or alternatively for one to increase while the other decreases and vice versa (negative correlation). The Spearman's rank correlation method is one of a number of methods which uses ranks in the analysis. For this reason they are known as *rank correlation* methods.

6.4.1 Rationale

Suppose that in a study six sets of paired measurements are made on two variables *X* and *Y* and the results ranked. If the ranking on the two scales is perfectly matched so that the same ranking is observed on both as shown in Table 6.4, the difference (d_i) in rank for each pair of observations will be zero. Therefore, the sum of the squared differences d_i^2 will equal zero too $(\Sigma d_i^2 = 0)$. In such a case one has perfect positive rank correlation. On the other hand, if the ranks are completely the other order for the two variables then the situation would be as shown in Table 6.5.

Table 6.4 Perfectly matched ranking.

Ranks							
X_i	1	2	3	4	5	6	
Y_i	1	2	3	4	5	6	
d_i	0	0	0	0	0	0	$\Sigma d_i = 0$
d_i^2	0	0	0	0	0	0	$\Sigma d_i^2 = 0$

Table 6.5 Completely opposite ranking.

Ranks							
X_i	1	2	3	4	5	6	
Y_i	6	5	4	3	2	1	
d_i	−5	−3	−1	1	3	5	$\Sigma d_i = 0$
d_i^2	25	9	1	1	9	25	$\Sigma d_i^2 = 70$

The sum of the squared differences Σd_i^2 would then be at its maximum. This maximum value can be calculated using the formula $(N^3 - N)/3$ where N = number of data pairs (six in this case). In such a case one has perfect negative rank correlation.

The Σd_i^2 value can be used as a test statistic. However, in the interest of ease of interpretation the test statistic is scaled so that when there is perfect positive rank correlation the correlation coefficient r_s is 1 and $r_s = -1$ when there is perfect negative rank correlation. This is achieved using the formula

$$r_s = 1 - \frac{6\sum d_i^2}{N^3 - 3} \tag{6.7}$$

Example 6.2

In a recent paper (Bowlt and Tiplady 1989) the authors investigated the possibility of a rank correlation between the iodine (^{129}I) radioactivity in individual thyroid glands and the distance of patients' homes from a nuclear power station (Sellafield). They reported an r_s value of −0.392 with $n = 130$.

Solution

To test whether this r_s value is significant, refer to Appendix 6. Since the sample size n is greater than 10, the t-statistic is used.

$$t = -0.392 \sqrt{\left[\frac{130 - 2}{1 - (-0.392)^2} \right]} = -4.82$$

This is an observation from the t-distribution with $(n-2)$ or 128 degrees of freedom under H_0. The critical value is -1.657 (see Appendix 2) for a lower one-tailed test at a significance level of 0.05. Therefore there appears to be a significant correlation between iodine radioactivity of the thyroid gland and the distance of the patients' homes from the nuclear plant. Indeed the significance probability is lower than 0.001.

6.4.2   *Tied observations*

When there are tied observations the mean rank is given to each observation in the set of ties and the equation given can be used without introducing serious error. However, when there are many ties the following correction factors should be used.

X_c, the correction factor for g ties in the X variable

$$= \sum_{j=1}^{g} \left(n_j^3 - n_j \right)$$

where n_i is the number of tied ranks in the jth grouping.

Y_c, the correction factor for ties in the Y variable is similarly calculated.

The formula for r_s is then defined by

$$r_s = \frac{\left(N^3 - N\right) - 6\sum d_i^2 - \left(X_c + Y_c\right)/2}{\sqrt{\left[\left(N^3 - N\right)^2 - \left(X_c + Y_c\right)\left(N^3 - N\right) + X_c Y_c\right]}} \tag{6.8}$$

6.4.3   *Caution*

- A strongly significant result does not imply a high correlation between the two variables considered and neither does a high correlation imply a strongly significant result. Spearman's rank correlation test simply assesses whether the data are consistent with the null hypothesis of zero correlation. A large n may render a small r_s value highly significant. Conversely with a small sample even a high r_s value may be consistent with H_0.
- The test statistic r_s measures the extent of monotonic (both variables changing in same direction) relationship between the two variables. Therefore although one may obtain an r_s value which may be very close to zero, one cannot say that there is no relationship between the two variables. There may well be a pronounced non-monotonic relationship. The best way to find out is to plot the data. Indeed such exploratory analysis should precede quantitative analysis as a matter of course.
- A high correlation does not imply a causal relationship (see Section 6.5 for a more thorough discussion).

6.5   Association and causation

If two variables are found to be associated, when can one conclude that there is a causal relationship between them? For example, if one observes an association between the aluminium content of drinking water and the incidence of senile dementia can one conclude that aluminium causes the disease?

Bradford-Hill (1965) has highlighted a number of important aspects to consider before deciding that the most likely interpretation of an association is causation:

(1) *Strength of association*:   For example, if exposure to a putative causative agent increases the incidence of a disease by a fraction, then the evidence in favour of a causal relationship would generally be viewed as being weaker than if the increase were several hundred-fold.

(2) *Consistency*:   If the association between two variables can be identified under different conditions, then the evidence in favour of causation is strengthened. For example, if the association between the aluminium content of drinking water and the incidence of senile dementia can be reproduced from country to country then the evidence in favour of a causal relationship is enhanced.

(3) *Specificity*:   The more specific the association, the more likely is the causal relationship. For example, a strong association between a pollutant and a rare disease provides stronger evidence in favour of a causal relationship than if a common disease was involved. The association between the acquired immunodeficiency syndrome (AIDS) and the homosexual community was highly specific and provided strong evidence in favour of the sexual transmission of the HIV virus. The danger in overstretching the conclusions and poorly defining the proposed cause and effect relationship can also be exemplified by considering AIDS. At one stage many were willing to exclude heterosexual sex as a possible means of developing AIDS.

(4) *Biological gradient*:   A significant Pearson's correlation coefficient will indicate a linear association between the two variables and hence provides evidence for a biological gradient.

The classical example here is the data showing a linear increase in death rate from cancer with the number of cigarettes smoked daily. An apparent biological gradient may, however, also be totally spurious. A recent example is the reported positive linear association between calcium intake and the incidence of hip fractures in different countries. Most of the other evidence indicates that the converse ought to be true, i.e. a negative correlation between the two variables.

(5) *Plausibility*:   If the association is supported by existing scientific knowledge about the two variables, the evidence in favour of a causal relationship is strengthened. For example, the knowledge that an agent causes cell mutation *in vitro* enhances the evidence supporting the theory that exposure to the agent increases the incidence of cancer. However, lack of such scientific plausibility should not by itself lead to rejection of a possible causal relation-

ship. Hence, the now widely accepted causal relationship between exposure to high-dose stilboestrol and ovarian cancer in the grandchildren was established before any biological plausibility became obvious. The same applied to the link between German measles during pregnancy and congenital malformations.

(6) *Temporal relationship*:   The exposure must precede the response. In practice this is often difficult to determine.

(7) *Coherence*:   The proposed causal relationship should not be contradicted by existing scientific knowledge about the disease. Conversely, scientific data may add to the coherence of the proposal. Identification of the HIV virus added much to the coherence of the proposed sexually transmitted nature of the virus.

6.6   Multiple linear regression

Very often the value which a response variable takes depends upon more than one independent variable. For example, the rate of a chemical reaction may depend both on temperature and pressure. Multiple linear regression enables us to test whether the independent variables do in fact alter the response through the use of an appropriate linear model. With such a model we are then able to make quantitative statements about the extent to which alterations in significant independent variables alter the response variable (e.g. how temperature and pressure affect the rate of a reaction). The errors associated with the estimates can also be defined.

6.6.1   The general multiple regression model

The general additive linear multiple regression model relating a dependent variable (Y) and k predictor variables ($X_1, X_2, \ldots, X_k$) takes the form

$$Y = \beta_0 + \beta_1 X_1 + \beta_2 X_2 + \ldots + \beta_k X_k + \varepsilon \qquad (6.9)$$

where ε, which represents the random variation, is normally distributed with mean 0 and variance σ^2 ($\varepsilon \sim N(0, \sigma^2)$).

The model implies that when the X variables are fixed at values $x_1, x_2, \ldots, x_k$, the mean value of Y given by $\bar{y}$ can be expressed by

$$\bar{y} = \beta_0 + \beta_1 x_1 + \beta_2 x_2 + \ldots + x_k \qquad (6.10)$$

The β values, ($\beta_0, \beta_1, \beta_2, \ldots, \beta_k$) are called the *population regression coefficients* and are estimated by *sample regression coefficients* ($b_0, b_1, b_2, \ldots, b_k$) as shown by the model

$$y = b_0 + b_1 x_1 + b_2 x_2 + \ldots + b_k x_k \qquad (6.11)$$

6.6.2   The polynomial regression model

In some instances the independent variables are all power terms of one single variable as shown below

$$y = \beta_0 + \beta_1 X_1 + \beta_2 X_1^2 + \ldots + \beta_k X_1^k + \varepsilon \tag{6.12}$$

Such a model, known as a *kth degree polynomial model*, can be rewritten in the form of the general multiple regression model (Equation 6.11)

$$y = \beta_0 + \beta_1 X_1 + \beta_2 X_2 + \ldots + \beta_k X_k + \varepsilon \tag{6.13}$$

where $X_2 = X_1^2, \ldots, X_k = X_1^k$.

6.6.3   The quadratic regression model

When only the X_1 and X_1^2 terms in Equation 6.12 are included, the reduced model is called a *quadratic regression model*.

6.6.4   Interaction between variables

Sometimes the change in the mean response ($\bar{y}$) associated with a given increase in one of the independent variables (X_1) depends on the value of a second variable (X_2). For example, the effect of temperature on a mean reaction rate may depend on the pressure. When this happens, we infer that there is interaction between X_1 and X_2. To model such an interaction a new variable X_3 is created, such that $X_3 = X_1 \times X_2$, for inclusion in the model

$$y = \beta_0 + B_1 X_1 + \beta_2 X_2 + \beta_3 X_1 X_2 + \varepsilon$$

or

$$y = \beta_0 + B_1 X_1 + \beta_2 X_2 + \beta_3 X_3 + \varepsilon \tag{6.14}$$

6.6.5   The full quadratic model

In many instances, cross-products of all the independent variables and other quadratic terms are included in the model. For example, for a model with two independent variables (X_1 and X_2), a possible model for the response y can be written as

$$y = \beta_0 + \beta_1 X_1 + \beta_2 X_2 + \beta_3 X_1 X_2 + \beta_4 X_1^2 + \beta_5 X_2^2 + \varepsilon$$

or

$$y = \beta_0 + \beta_1 X_1 + \beta_2 X_2 + \beta_3 X_3 + \beta_4 X_4 + \beta_5 X_5 + \varepsilon$$

Such a model is called a full quadratic model and is widely used in a technique called *surface response modelling*.

6.6.6 Multiple linear regression with categorical variables

In addition to being useful for modelling continuous variables, multiple linear regression may also be used with categorical independent variables. For example, the lung function (y) of a person may be described by the model

$$y = \beta_0 + \beta_1 \left(Age \right) + \beta_2 \left(Sex \right) + \varepsilon$$

or

$$y = \beta_0 + \beta_1 X_1 + \beta_2 X_2 + \varepsilon \tag{6.15}$$

X_1 representing age, is a continuous variable. The variable X_2, for sex of the individual, is however a categorical variable. To incorporate it into the model, X_2 is introduced as a *dummy variable* which can only take two values as shown:

$$X_2 = \begin{cases} 1 \text{ if male} \\ 0 \text{ if female} \end{cases}$$

Q6.1

How would you proceed if you wanted to test for the significance of previous history of asthma, hay fever and bronchitis in your lung function model (Equation 6.15)?

A6.1

It may be tempting to include a variable taking three values (e.g. 1 for asthma, 2 for hay fever and 3 for bronchitis). This would be wrong since it assumes an ordering of the categories which may not be there. The solution is to use two dummy variables as shown

$$X_3 = \begin{cases} 1 \text{ if asthma} \\ 0 \text{ otherwise} \end{cases} \qquad X_4 = \begin{cases} 1 \text{ if bronchitis} \\ 0 \text{ otherwise} \end{cases}$$

A patient with bronchitis is then represented by $(X_3 = X_4 = 0)$.

In general if it is required to include a categorical variable with k categories, $(k - 1)$ dummy variables will be required.

6.6.7 Assessing the value of a model

$$Y = \beta_0 + \beta_1 X_1 + \beta_2 X_2 + \ldots + \beta_k X_k + \varepsilon \tag{6.9}$$

Data on $X_1, X_2, \ldots, X_k$ and Y are collected and fitted to the model. This is done by minimising the sum of the squared deviations (SSE) between the observed Y values and the values predicted by the model

$$Y = b_0 + b_1 X_1 + b_2 X_2 + \ldots + b_k X_k$$

$$\text{SSE} = \sum \left(y_i - \left[b_0 + b_1 x_1 + b_2 x_2 + \ldots + b_k x_k \right] \right)^2 \tag{6.16}$$

The calculations are tedious and are usually done by computer to yield b_0, b_1, $b_2, \ldots, b_k$ values. The usefulness of the model is determined by how close the predicted Y values are to the observed values.

To illustrate the use of multiple linear regression Example 6.3 will be analysed using the computer package MINITAB and SAS. The matrix manipulations necessary for illustrating the calculations are beyond the scope of this book. The following discussion will therefore emphasise the interpretation of the computer outputs and the hypothesis tests which can be carried out using the statistics displayed.

Example 6.3

A study by Schultz (1987) used octanol-water partition coefficient (P) and ionisation constant (Ka) to model the toxicity of phenols. The response was the logarithm of the concentration of the phenol required to inhibit the growth of a microorganism by 50% compared to a control. The model proposed was of the form

$$\log \text{Response} = \alpha + \beta_1 (\log P) + \beta_2 (pKa) + \varepsilon \tag{6.17}$$

where pKa is the logarithm of the ionisation constant to base 10.

Solution

Table 6.6 reproduces the values reported by Schultz. LogRes1 refers to the logarithm of the response, LogP1 to the logarithm of the partition coefficient and pKa1 to the pKa value.

Table 6.6 Biological and physico-chemical data on a series of phenolic compounds.

LogRes1	LogP1	pKa1
−1.043	0.49	9.74
−0.652		
−0.143		

MINITAB Commands

	Objective
`MTB>Regress C1 2 C2 C3;`	This asks MINITAB to perform a regression of data stored in column 1 (LogRes1) with two independent variables (LogP1 and pKa1) stored in columns 2 and 3.
`MTB>Predict 2, 9.5.`	This asks MINITAB to predict the LogRes1 value corresponding to LogP1 = 2 and pKa1 = 9.5.

MINITAB output

```
The regression equation is
LogRes1 = 0.819 + 0.567 LogP1 - 0.189 pKa1

Predictor          Coef        Stdev       t-ratio           p
Constant         0.8190       0.2385          3.43       0.003
LogP1            0.56709      0.03593        15.78       0.000
pKa1            -0.18852      0.02270        -8.30       0.000

s = 0.2253      R-sq = 95.8%      R-sq(adj) = 95.3%

Analysis of Variance

SOURCE          DF           SS          MS            F           P
Regression       2       20.847      10.423       205.29       0.000
Error           18        0.914       0.051
Total           20       21.761

SOURCE        DF       SEQ SS
LogP1          1       17.346
pKa1           1        3.500

Unusual Observations
Obs.    LogP1    LogRes1        Fit    Stdev.Fit     Residual     St.Resid
21       5.68     2.6640     3.1691       0.1212      -0.5051        -2.66R

R denotes an obs. with a large st. resid.

   Fit   Stdev.Fit        95% C.I.              95% P.I.
0.1622      0.0627    (0.0304, 0.2941)    (-0.3293, 0.6538)
```

Q6.2
In the output, identify the coefficients α, β_1 and β_2.

A6.2
$\alpha = 0.8190$ $\beta_1 = 0.56709$ $\beta_2 = -0.18852$

Q6.3
How much of the sum of squares is explained by the regression model?

A6.3
95.8%.   This is given by the R^2 value. Remember $R^2 = (SSRegression)/(SSTotal) = (SSReg)/(SSTo)$.

Q6.4
Carry out the hypothesis test

$H_0 : \beta_1 = \beta_2 = 0$
$H_1 :$ at least one of β_1 and β_2 is not zero.

A6.4

From the computer output

The test statistic = MSRegression/MSResidual = MSReg/MSE
$$= 10.4235/0.0508 = 205.29$$

This is a statistic from the $F_{1,19}$ distribution. At a significance probability of 0.05, the critical value is 5.98 (Neave, 1979). Therefore H_0 is rejected.

Q6.5

Carry out the hypothesis test

$H_0 : \beta_1 = 0$
$H_1 : \beta_1 \neq 0$

A6.5

The test statistic is, from the computer output

$$t' = b_i / s_{b_i} = b_1 / s_{b_1} = \frac{0.56709}{0.03593} = 15.78$$

This is a statistic from the t-distribution with $(N - n - 1)$ degrees of freedom (df) or $(20 - 2)$ or 18 df.
   At a significance probability of 0.05, the critical value is 2.10 (Appendix 2). Therefore H_0 can be rejected and H_1 accepted.

Q6.6

Carry out the hypothesis test

$H_0 : \beta_1 = 0$
$H_1 : \beta_1 \neq 0$

A6.6

Using the same approach as Q6.5 above

$$t' = b_2 / s_{b_2} = \frac{-0.18852}{0.02270} = -8.30$$

and H_0 can again be rejected.

Q6.7

Calculate the 95% confidence interval (CI) for the estimates of β_1 and β_2 (see Chapter 12).

A6.7

$$95\% \text{ CI} = b_i \pm [t_{0.975}] \times s_{b_i}$$
$$\therefore \quad 95\% \text{ CI for } b_1 = 0.56709 \pm [2.10] \times 0.03593$$
$$= [0.492, \ 0.643]$$
$$95\% \text{ CI for } b_2 = -0.18852 \pm [2.10] \times 0.02270$$
$$= [-0.236, \ -0.141]$$

Q6.8

What do the values $\beta_1 = 0.567$ and $\beta_2 = -0.189$ mean?

A6.8

The $\beta_1 = 0.567$ value indicates that it is estimated that the logResponse value will increase by 0.567 unit whenever the logP value increases by one unit and the pKa value is held constant. Similarly the value $\beta_2 = -0.189$ value is an estimate of how much the logResponse value will increase for every unit increase in pKa and logP is held constant.

Q6.9

When modelling data it is important not to add more variables than is necessary. Does adding the pKa variable improve the simple linear model

$$\log \text{Response} = \alpha + \beta_1 (\log P) + \varepsilon$$

A6.9

Simple linear regression gives the following equation

$$\log \text{Response} = -0.929 + 0.643 \log P1$$

with an R^2 value of 79.7% and an F-value of 74.66.

   Since adding the independent variable (pKa) increases the percentage of the sum of squares explained by the regression model from 79.7% to 95.8%, the addition appears to be useful in providing a better model for the data. However note that addition of an additional independent variable will always increase the R^2 value. Therefore it is important to adjust for any additional variable included in the model. To do this, the formula

$$R^2_{\text{adjusted}} = 1 - \left(\frac{n-1}{n-k} \right) \frac{\text{SSE}}{\text{SSTo}} \tag{6.18}$$

is used where n is the number of observations and k is the number of independent variables. Using this statistic, the R^2_{adjusted} values are 95.3% for the two independent variables model and 78.6% for the one independent variable model (see computer outputs). Therefore the tentative conclusion that the additional variable improves the model holds.

Q6.10

One of the possible problems with multiple regression analysis arises from *collinearity*, that is when the independent variables are correlated. When this is the case, it is not possible to attribute the change observed in the response *uniquely* to any of the correlated independent variables. Is this a problem with the pKa and logP data?

A6.10

Correlation analysis between logP and pKa gives an R^2 value of 6.4% and regression analysis gives an F-value of 1.30 in the $F_{1,19}$ distribution. The probability of that F-value in this distribution is 0.269. Therefore, collinearity does not seem to be a significant problem in the model used.

Q6.11
Calculate the predicted mean LogRes1 when LogP1 = 2 and pKa1 = 9.5 and give the corresponding 95% confidence interval.

A6.11
The predicted mean LogRes1 is obtained by substituting the appropriate value into the regression equation.

$$LogRes1 = 0.8190 + 0.56709 \times (2)\ 0.18852 \times (9.5)$$
$$= 0.1622$$

The associated 95% confidence interval is given by

$$\text{Predicted Mean [LogRes1] value} \pm [t_{0.975}] \times SE(\text{of LogRes1})$$

or

$$0.1622 \pm 2.101 \times 0.0627 = [0.030,\ 0.294].$$

This is the same as the output obtained by using the predict subcommand in the MINITAB session. See the last lines of the output.

Q6.12
The output on the last line also includes a 95% PI. What is it?

A6.12
The 95% PI refers to the 95% prediction interval for an individual LogRes1 value. In the example used the range [–0.3293, 0.6538] gives the 95% confidence interval for a single LogRes1 value when LogP1 = 2 and pKa1 = 9.5.

SAS commands
```
data test;

infile 'a:phenol.dat';
input logP1 pKa1 logRes1;
run;
proc print;
run;
proc reg;
model logRes1 = logP1 pKa1 / p r cli clm;
run;
```

SAS output
```
Model: MODEL1
Dependent Variable: LOGRES1
```

Analysis of Variance

Source	DF	Sum of Squares	Mean Square	F Value	Prob > F
Model	2	20.84689	10.42345	205.294	0.0001
Error	18	0.91392	0.05077		
C Total	20	21.76081			

Root MSE	0.22533	R-square	0.9580
Dep Mean	0.93243	Adj R-sq	0.9533
C.V.	24.16583		

Parameter Estimates

Variable	DF	Parameter Estimate	Standard Error	T for H0: Parameter = 0	Prob > |T|
INTERCEP	1	0.819025	0.23850248	3.434	0.0030
LOGP1	1	0.567093	0.03592909	15.784	0.0001
PKA1	1	-0.188523	0.02270486	-8.303	0.0001

Obs	Dep Var LOGRES1	Predict Value	Std Err Predict	Lower95% Mean	Upper95% Mean	Lower95% Predict	Upper95% Predict
1	-1.0430	-0.7393	0.098	-0.9457	-0.5330	-1.2557	-0.2229
2	-0.6520	-0.5767	0.090	-0.7659	-0.3875	-1.0865	-0.0669
3	-0.1430	-0.3044	0.078	-0.4693	-0.1395	-0.8057	0.1969
4	-0.0650	0.1599	0.064	0.0246	0.2952	-0.3325	0.6523
5	0.1920	0.00191	0.070	-0.1462	0.1500	-0.4941	0.4979
6	0.2770	0.4377	0.056	0.3208	0.5546	-0.0499	0.9253
7	-0.0290	0.1288	0.074	-0.0257	0.2833	-0.3692	0.6267
8	0.2060	0.3969	0.064	0.2618	0.5320	-0.0954	0.8892
9	0.7950	0.6349	0.059	0.5113	0.7584	0.1456	1.1241
10	1.0360	1.0801	0.050	0.9756	1.1846	0.5953	1.5649
11	1.0940	0.9241	0.064	0.7907	1.0575	0.4322	1.4159
12	1.2330	1.1381	0.089	0.9511	1.3251	0.6291	1.6471
13	1.6480	1.5802	0.097	1.3774	1.7830	1.0652	2.0952
14	2.0330	1.9545	0.116	1.7118	2.1972	1.4225	2.4865
15	0.9290	0.8274	0.099	0.6194	1.0353	0.3103	1.3444
16	1.0960	1.1387	0.117	0.8931	1.3842	0.6054	1.6720
17	1.7500	1.3907	0.080	1.2218	1.5596	0.8881	1.8934
18	1.6310	1.4725	0.064	1.3380	1.6069	0.9804	1.9646
19	2.3610	2.0503	0.084	1.8744	2.2263	1.5453	2.5554
20	2.5680	2.7157	0.102	2.5018	2.9296	2.1962	3.2352
21	2.6640	3.1691	0.121	2.9145	3.4238	2.6316	3.7067

Comments on SAS output

Note that the analysis of variance table is the same as that obtained with MINITAB as are the parameter estimates. The adequacy of the model is tested by the analysis of variance. MINITAB prints out the regression equation and this makes interpretation easier. The 95% confidence intervals (CI) and the 95% prediction intervals (PI) are also given for all observations.

Subcommands under the Regression command also enable a whole host of other statistics to be computed with SAS.

6.7 Caution

When an overall model is analysed by multiple linear regression and it is found that the regression explained by the model is significant, care must be exercised in interpreting this result. In particular, the model postulated may not be the only, or indeed the most appropriate, model for explaining the data. Insight which the investigator has into the scientific problem being investigated should be used to propose alternative, and the most rational, models.

6.8 Non-linear regression

In linear regression the equations being fitted are linear in the parameters. With many systems of interest to the health scientist, the models are non-linear with respect to the parameters. Many rate processes, for example, follow exponential kinetics of the form

$$Y = Ae^{-kt} \tag{6.19}$$

where Y is the response, t is the independent variable and A and k are constants or parameters describing the reactions. Similarly, growth equations commonly take the form described by the logistic equation:

$$Y = A/\left(1 - ke^{-Bt}\right) \tag{6.20}$$

where A, k and B are the parameters and Y and t the variables.

Equations such as 6.19 can be linearised by appropriate transformations. For example, Equation 6.19 can be transformed into the following linear equation:

$$\text{Log}_e\left(Y\right) = \log_e\left(A\right) - kt \tag{6.21}$$

The transformed Y values can then be fitted using the standard linear regression approach.

In other cases, such as with the logistic equation (Equation 6.20), transformation into an equation linear in the parameters cannot be done and methods collectively known as non-linear regression must be used.

6.8.1 What then is non-linear regression

Non-linear regression is a procedure for fitting data to equations which are non-linear in the parameters. As with linear regression, the objective is to determine values of parameters which ensure that the given non-linear equation most closely approximates the observations obtained. This is most commonly done by minimising the residual sum of squares (SSE).

Unlike linear regression which solves the problem in one step, in non-linear regression, an iterative approach is used. In other words, a set of initial estimates for the parameters are fed in and the SSE calculated. The values are then progressively altered using an appropriate algorithm (procedure) to reduce the SSE until a minimum is achieved. Various algorithms are commonly used for this purpose, including the Gauss-Newton, the method of steepest descent and the Marquardt algorithms. A mathematical description of those iterative procedures is beyond the scope of this book.

6.8.2 Points to note

- To perform a non-linear regression on a set of data one must therefore have a model which one hopes will describe the data. Non-linear regression does not identify the best form of equation to use. It simply optimises the parameters *given* an equation. Insight into the problem being investigated is therefore essential.

- A set of initial estimates for the parameters is required. This is obtained intelligently by guesswork using the literature and the data available. For example, initial rates and terminal rates are often useful for obtaining quick initial estimates of parameters in kinetic work.

  Good initial estimates are required to ensure convergence to a solution and more appropriately convergence to the correct minimum, commonly referred to as local minima because they are the minimum values in the regions defined by the poor initial estimates.

- Convergence is achieved when the SSE reaches a level defined by the user. Again knowledge of the problem to hand is invaluable for making the appropriate judgement.

- Unless data are appropriately scaled nonsensical estimates may be obtained. For example, round off errors may yield invalid estimates if values are entered as $0-10^{15}$. Scaling to a 1–10 scale would overcome such problems. This of course applies to other calculations too but falling into this trap is more common with users of non-linear regression.

- Obtaining the best parameter estimates by minimisation of the sum of squares assumes that the errors associated with the y values are independent of the size of those values. This is commonly not the case since in many studies some measurements are done close to the sensitivity of the equipment, and the errors are higher with those values than with others. In such a case weighting is used.

Various weighting schemes are commonly used. For example, the deviation of each point from the curve may be divided by the y response at that point and squared. Ensure that the y values are within the domain of the weighting function. For example, if the reciprocal of y is used then zero values are not appropriate since the weighting function is then indeterminate.

- To evaluate how good the fit obtained is, a plot of the proposed curve superimposed on the data is usually highly illuminating. A plot of the residuals often reveals poor fits which the first plot fails to bring up. A good fit should be associated with randomly distributed errors.

The sum of the squared residuals divided by the degrees of freedom gives the mean variance of the curve from the points. This is referred to as the mean square error (MSE). The square root of that term gives the standard deviation of the curve from the points and is referred to as the root mean square error (RMSE). One's objective is to obtain as low a value for the RMSE as possible. Examining the RMSE is particularly useful when comparing alternative models which make equal scientific sense.

If the competing models have the same number of parameters, then a straight comparison of the MSE is sufficient. The ratio is distributed according to the F-distribution with $(N - k)$ degrees of freedom where N is the number of points and k the number of parameters being investigated.

Increasing the number of parameters will usually improve the fit. Therefore this must be accounted for when making comparison of alternative models. The test statistic used is given by

$$F = \frac{\left(\text{SSE1} - \text{SSE2}\right)\big/\left(k_1 - k_2\right)}{\text{SSE}_2/k_2} \tag{6.22}$$

where k_1 and k_2 are the parameters associated with models 1 and 2 and SSE1 and SSE2 are the corresponding residual sums of squares. The statistic follows an F-distribution with $(k_1 - k_2)$ and k_2 degrees of freedom.

The r^2 value, the square of the correlation coefficient, gives the fraction of the total variance of the y values. A perfect fit, as with linear regression, gives an r^2 value of unity and an r^2 value of 0 shows total lack of fit.

- One common research question is whether the parameters of a particular process have altered with a change in experimental conditions. For example, the blood level (Y) profile of an orally ingested drug often follows a time (t) course described by an equation of the form

$$Y = \text{Ae}^{-k_1 t} + \text{Be}^{-k_2 t} \tag{6.23}$$

where A, k_1 and k_2 are parameters to be estimated.

One experiment may involve measuring those parameters under controlled conditions and under alkaline urinary conditions. The question posed is whether the rate constants have changed. One approach is to carry out three sets of estimates, the first with the data for the control run, the second with the data from the test run (alkaline urine) and the third with the two sets of pooled data. Three error sum of squares, SSE1, SSE2 and SSEP (pooled), are obtained. The test statistic

$$F = \frac{(SSEP - SSE12)/(n_p - n_{12})}{SSE12/n_{12}}$$

(6.24)

is calculated where SSE12 = SSE1 + SSE2 and $n_{12} = n_1 + n_2$, the sum of the degrees of freedom associated with the error terms in the first and second runs respectively.

The test statistic is then referred to the F-distribution with $(n_p - n_{12})$ and n_{12} degrees of freedom for an appropriate F-test (see Chapters 2 and 7).

- It is often possible to express a given non-linear equation in several forms. This process, called *reparameterisation*, may be required to obtain convergence, particularly with highly non-linear equations with many parameters. The objective is to convert the equation to one which is as close as possible to one which is linear.

6.8.3   Computer programs

MINITAB can be used to carry out non-linear regression using a macro written by Stork (1990). The Gauss-Newton method is used. SAS uses the procedure NLIN to perform non-linear regression. A wide range of algorithms is included. Example 6.4 illustrates the calculation of a non-linear regression.

Example 6.4
Example 6.4 deals with an investigation of the breakdown of aspirin in solution as a function of time. The data in Table 6.7 show the concentration of aspirin as a function of time.

Table 6.7   Data held in a MINITAB worksheet on the breakdown of aspirin in solution.

Aspmg	558	516	489	450	427	400	374	348	308	272	240	212	186	162	145
Timemim	18	35	51	68	85	101	118	136	166	197	229	260	292	326	355
Init Par	600	−0.004													

The variable Aspmg refers to the amount of aspirin remaining in solution in mg. The variable Timemin refers to time in minutes. The Aspmg and Timemin data are paired. InitPar refers to initial parameter estimates for A and k (see Equation 6.19).

General approach to non-linear regression
When using a non-linear regression program one needs to specify the model or equation to which the data are to be fitted, initial estimates of the parameters concerned and the iterative procedure to be used when several options are available. The MINITAB macro mentioned above uses the Gauss-Newton method while SAS provides a number of procedures. Two of

them, the Gauss-Newton and the Marquardt methods will be discussed. Both methods require the partial derivatives of the response variable with respect to the parameters. Some specialist programs use difference equations to approximate the partial derivatives and appear to function as well.

The model
$$y = \alpha e^{kt} + \varepsilon \tag{6.25}$$

where y = amount of aspirin remaining (Aspmg), t is the time in minutes (Time min), α and β are the parameters to be estimated and ε is a normally distributed error term with mean 0.

The partial derivatives
$$\partial y / \partial \alpha = e^{kt} \quad \text{and} \quad \partial y / \partial k = \alpha k e^{kt} \tag{6.26}$$

The initial estimates
$\alpha = 600$ from a knowledge of approximate concentration of the initial solution and $k = 0.004$ from a linear regression on the following equation $\log_e y = \log \alpha + kt$.

MINITAB output
The output obtained with five iterations is shown below:

```
Final iteration number, parameter estimates, and SSE:
K15      5.00000


Row      gk           SSE

1        596.839      52.9008
2        -0.004


Estimated approximate variance-covariance matrix of the parameters:
MATRIX M11

 1.8712450    -0.0000202
-0.0000202     0.0000000
```

The residual sum of squares (SSE) are somewhat high and a plot of the residuals indeed showed a downward trend with time suggesting that an alternative model may be required or some of the early or late points are poor. In this case a knowledge of solution kinetics suggests that the latter interpretation is more likely (see under SAS output 1 below).

SAS commands
The following SAS program produced the SAS output 1 shown below.

	Objective
`data a;`	Label.
`infile 'a:test3.dat';`	Locates data set.
`input y t;`	Inputs y and t.
`run;`	

```
proc print;                                      Prints input data.
run;
proc NLIN method = Gauss                         Calls non-linear regression routine.
Parms A0 = 600                                   Initial estimates.
     k1 = -0.04;
model y = A0*Exp(k1*t);                           Model.
der.A0 = Exp(k1*t);                               Partial derivatives.
der.k1 = A0 Exp(k1*t);
output out = b p = yhat r = yresid;               Output sought.
proc plot data = b;                               Plot of data and results.
plot y*t = 'A' yhat*t = 'E' /overlay vpos = 25;
plot yresid*t / vref = 0 vpos = 25;
run;
```

SAS output 1

```
              Non-Linear Least Squares Iterative Phase
              Dependent Variable Y Method: Gauss-Newton


    Iter            A0                 k1            Sum of Squares
     0          600.000000         -0.040000            1468687
     1          398.844690         -0.017179            1114023
     2          362.941947         -0.003852             291708
     3          596.771735         -0.004067          246.441931
     4          596.810995         -0.003984           52.917756
     5          596.839091         -0.003985           52.900753
     6          596.839073         -0.003985           52.900753
NOTE: Convergence criterion met.


 Non-Linear Least Squares Summary Statistics    Dependent Variable Y


   Source                 DF       Sum of Squares        Mean Square

   Regression              2       1975754.0992        987877.0496
   Residual               13            52.9008             4.0693
   Uncorrected Total      15       1975807.0000

   (Corrected Total)      14        250635.7333


Parameter      Estimate      Asymptotic              Asymptotic 95%
                             Std. Error           Confidence Interval
                                                  Lower          Upper
    A0      596.8390728    1.3679335821    593.88383371    599.79431184
    k1       -0.0039852    0.0000188973     -0.00402607     -0.00394442
```

SAS output 1 also gives a plot of predicted and observed values as well as a plot of residuals. By replacing the word Gauss by Marquardt in the SAS program, the Marquardt procedure is used to produce SAS output 2.

SAS output 2

```
          Non-Linear Least Squares Iterative Phase
          Dependent Variable Y Method: Marquardt

   Iter          A0              k1          Sum of Squares
    0        600.000000      -0.040000           1468687
    1        682.183960      -0.032044           1261703
    2        831.464845      -0.007227            102552
    3        559.408093      -0.003732         3874.259190
    4        596.589080      -0.003992           55.764216
    5        596.838726      -0.003985           52.900755
    6        596.839073      -0.003985           52.900753
    7        596.839073      -0.003985           52.900753
NOTE: Convergence criterion met.
```

Interpreting SAS outputs

Examination of the SAS output indicates that the residual sum of squares is rather high, in agreement with the MINITAB output. To check the adequacy of the model examine the residual plot shown in Fig. 6.6.

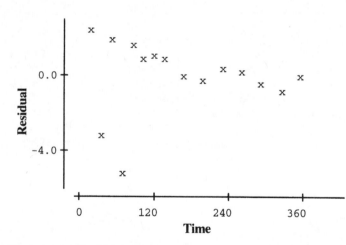

Fig. 6.6   Residual plot for aspirin data.

This shows that two of the points seem to be outliers. Chemical reanalysis of the solutions indicates that the values for aspirin concentration at times 35 and 68 minutes should have been 521 and 450. The new values were used and the residual plot shown in Fig. 6.7 was obtained. This showed that the data now fit the model very well. The residual sum of squares was reduced to 1.35 from 52.9 and the residuals are evenly distributed around zero.

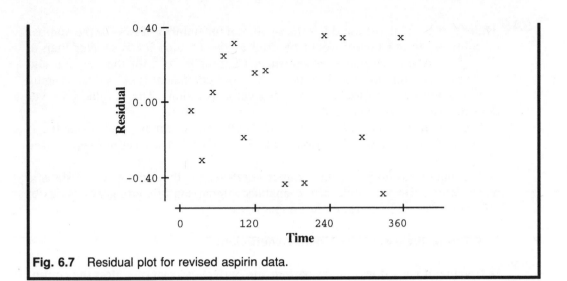

Fig. 6.7   Residual plot for revised aspirin data.

6.9   Other correlation methods

6.9.1   *Cramér coefficient, C*

The Cramér coefficient, C, is a measure of the extent of association between sets of variables. It is particularly useful for analysing categorical data cast in the form of contingency tables (see Chapter 9) such as the one shown in Table 6.8.

Table 6.8   Layout for a $k \times k$ contingency table.

		Variable set 1				
		x_1	x_2	...	...	x_k
	y_1	n_{11}	n_{12}	...	...	n_{1k}
	y_2	n_{21}	n_{22}	...	...	n_{2k}
Variable set 2	:	:				
	:	:				
	y_j	n_{j1}	n_{j2}	...	...	n_{jk}

If $N = n_{11} + n_{12} + \ldots + n_{jk}$, the total number of counts in the contingency table then the Cramér coefficient, C, is given by

$$C = \sqrt{\left[\frac{\chi^2}{N(L-1)} \right]} \qquad (6.27)$$

where χ^2 is the χ^2 statistic and L is the smaller of the number of rows or the number of columns. In our table j would be used as the L value if j is smaller than k. The χ^2 statistic is calculated as shown in Chapter 9. As with the Pearson and Spearman's correlation coefficients, the Cramér coefficient takes values ranging from 0 (independent variables) to 1 (perfect association). The C value however does not take negative values.

The significance of an observed Cramér coefficient, C, can be tested using the χ^2 test with reference to the χ^2 distribution with $(j-1)(k-1)$ degrees of freedom (see Chapter 9).

One major advantage of the Cramér coefficient is that unlike the χ^2 statistic which is sensitive to sample size, it enables comparison of contingency tables of different sizes based on different sample sizes.

Caution in the use of the Cramér coefficient

A C value of unity does not always indicate perfect association unless the contingency table is square. When the number of columns exceeds the number of rows, a C value of 1 indicates perfect column to row association but not vice versa. Similarly when the number of rows exceeds the number of columns, a C value of one shows perfect row to column variation only.

The sample sizes must be large, typically with no more than one fifth of the cells having expected frequencies smaller than 5 and no cell having an expected frequency of less than one. These are the conditions applicable when the χ^2 test is used.

The C^2 value has no equivalent meaning to that of the Pearson r^2 value which represents the proportion of the total variances accounted for by the relationship.

6.9.2   The phi coefficient, r_ϕ

The phi coefficient, r_ϕ, is used as a measure of the extent of association between dichotomous variables (categorical with only two possible outcomes each). In practice its use is usually restricted to the analysis of 2×2 contingency tabular data (see Chapter 9).

Consider the contingency table given in Table 6.9. The phi coefficient r_ϕ is calculated using equation

Table 6.9 Lay-out of a 2×2 contingency table. All entries are counts not percentages or fractions.

	Variable X 1	2	Total count
Variable Y 1	n_a	n_b	$n_a + n_b$
2	n_c	n_d	$n_c + n_d$
Total count	$n_a + n_c$	$n_b + n_d$	$n_a + n_b + n_c + n_d$

$$r_\phi = \frac{\left|n_a n_d - n_b n_c\right|}{\sqrt{\left[\left(n_a + n_c\right)\left(n_b + n_d\right)\left(n_a + n_b\right)\left(n_c + n_d\right)\right]}}$$ (6.28)

For a 2×2 contingency table, r_ϕ can range from 0 to 1 depending on how strong the association is. The significance of r_ϕ is tested using the χ^2 test (large samples) or the Fisher's exact test (small samples) (see Chapter 9).

6.9.3 Kendall's rank correlation coefficient, τ

Kendall's rank correlation coefficient (τ or tau) is used in the same way as Spearman's correlation coefficient in that both are measures of association between two variables which are measured in at least an ordinal scale. Each unit under study produces a pair of observations (x_i, y_i) with respect to the two variables (x and y).

The statistic is calculated by comparing all possible pairs of (x, y) values with each other. If all the (x_i, y_i) values have the same rank order then $\tau = 1$. If the ranks are completely reversed then $\tau = -1$.

Tau (τ) can be calculated as shown in Fig. 6.8.

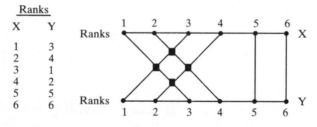

Fig. 6.8   Plot of ranked data.

Step 1
Rank the observations and tabulate as shown in Fig. 6.8.

Step 2
Plot as shown in Fig. 6.8. The ranks can be replaced by actual values if an interval scale is used.

Step 3
Count the number of discordant (N_D) pairs of observations given by the number of intersections (■); four in the example above.

Step 4

$$\tau = 1 - \frac{4N_D}{n(n-1)}$$ (6.29)

where n is the number of pairs of observations.

$$\tau = 1 - \frac{4 \times 4}{6(6-1)}$$

$= 0.47$ in Fig. 6.8.

Testing the significance of observed τ

The observed τ statistic can be referred to a table such as Appendix 12 to evaluate its significance.

Dealing with ties

Suppose that the observations shown in Fig. 6.9 were made. These can be plotted graphically as shown below. Note that proper scaling is unnecessary. It can be shown that there are two discordant pairs. As they intersect on the X or Y axes, indicating ties, they are given a 0.5 score each. Kendall's tau is then given by

$$\tau = 1 - \frac{4(2 \times 0.5)}{7 \times 6} = 0.9048$$

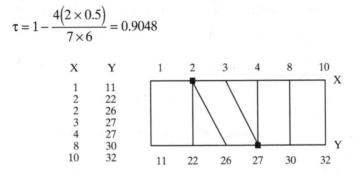

Fig. 6.9   Plot of ranked data with ties.

6.9.4   *Kendall's coefficient of concordance, W*

In many studies there is a need to compare more than two sets of rankings of N experimental units (objects or individuals) to test whether the rankings agree with each other. Kendall's coefficient of concordance, W, is used as such a measure of association or concordance between the different sets of rankings. If there is concordance in the rankings, the pooled ranking may be used as a standard. There is no guarantee that the ordering is necessarily correct even in the presence of a highly significant coefficient W.

6.9.5   *Kendall's partial rank correlation coefficient*

When it is suspected that a third variable may contribute to the association seen between two variables and there is no satisfactory way of maintaining the third variable constant during the study, one may then resort to *statistical control* by using partial correlation techniques. Analysis of covariance is such a technique when the response is numerical and precise specific parametric assumptions are met (see Chapter 8). Kendall's partial rank correlation method is a non-parametric method for exercising statistical control.

6.9.6   Kendall's coefficient of agreement, U

In some studies the experimental units (objects or individuals) are paired with replacement. Each judge is then asked to rank the units included within each pair and by so-doing indicates a preference. For example, with four experimental units (A, B, C, D), there are six possible comparisons ($^4C_2$) as shown: AB AC AD BC BD CD. The preferences of one judge could be A A D C D C. Kendall's coefficient of agreement, U, is used as a measure of agreement among judges in their preferences in such paired comparison studies.

6.9.7   The Kappa statistic, κ

The Kappa statistic is used as a measure of agreement between several judges' assignments of experimental units to a set of categories which cannot be ordered. This is quite distinct from Kendall's coefficient of agreement (U) and Kendall's coefficient of concordance (W) which require ordinal data. Several types of Kappa statistics are in common use (see Cohen, 1960, 1968; Fleiss, 1971; Landis and Koch, 1977).

6.9.8   The Gamma statistic, γ

The Gamma statistic is used for measuring the relationship between two ordinally-scaled variables and is particularly useful when there are many ties and the data can be cast in the form of a contingency table (see Chapter 9). The Spearman's rank order correlation coefficient and Kendall's rank order correlation coefficient are less appropriate in the presence of many ties.

If the variables are independent the gamma statistic $\gamma = 0$. If there are no disagreements in the rankings $\gamma = 1$ and if there are no agreements $\gamma = -1$ (see Goodman and Kruskal, 1954, 1972).

6.9.9   The Iman-Conover method

The Iman-Conover method is a non-parametric regression method that assumes only that the relationship between the two variables studied is monotonic (i.e. both variables changing in the same direction).

The non-parametric methods discussed in this chapter are discussed in detail by Siegel and Castellan (1988) and Neave (1988). Non-linear regression techniques are considered by Ratkowsky (1989) and Bates (1988).

Chapter 7
Hypothesis Testing About More Than Two Populations

7.1 Analysis of variance (ANOVA)

Analysis of variance is a method developed by R.A. Fisher (1890–1962) to deal with the fact that if one carries out a set of hypothesis tests, each at a given significance level (α_1), the experimentwise (α) level is not α_1 but some larger value which depends on the number of comparisons made. The rationale underlying analysis of variance (ANOVA) is elegantly simple. Fisher reasoned that if the total variability in the data of interest could be partitioned into additive components, that is variability due to random variation and to the factors under investigation, then by taking appropriate ratios (*F*-ratio), one ought to be able to determine whether there are true differences in the parameter of interest in the populations concerned. Fisher worked out the probability distributions for those ratios thereby enabling the calculation of the probability of occurrence of any given ratio. The *F*-ratio and the rationale behind ANOVA is further discussed below. Figure 7.1 provides a flow chart to illustrate where ANOVA fits in the range of hypothesis tests when dealing with samples from more than two populations.

7.1.1 One factor ANOVA

In one-factor ANOVA one is concerned with one dependent (response) variable and one independent variable. Examples of cases when one-factor ANOVA is appropriate are:

(1) Experiments in which subjects are randomly allocated to receive one of a number of treatments and the mean responses are compared.
(2) Comparison of the mean vitamin C content of different varieties of tomatoes grown under the same conditions.
(3) Comparison of the mean birth weights of babies of mothers who are smokers, ex-smokers and non-smokers, in an otherwise homogeneous population of mothers.

7.1.2 Rationale

To illustrate the rationale behind ANOVA suppose that the data in Table 7.1 were collected on the vitamin C content (mg/100 g) of samples of three different varieties of tomatoes.

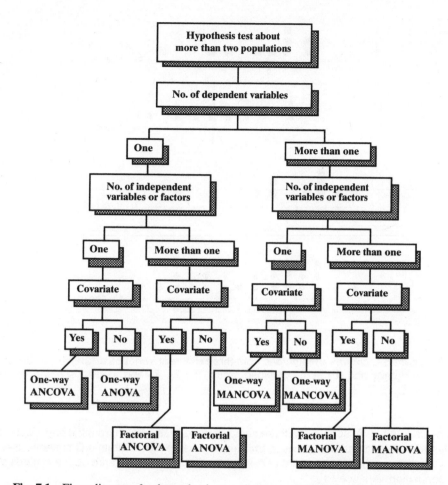

Fig. 7.1   Flow diagram for hypothesis test about more than two populations.

Table 7.1   Vitamin C content of three varieties of tomatoes.

Variety of tomato	Vitamin C (mg/100 g)
1	26, 18, 22, 23, 17, 18, 19, 17, 18, 20
2	23, 18, 25, 27, 24, 23, 18, 22, 25, 21
3	25, 20, 16, 14, 17, 19, 16, 15, 16, 19

Example 7.1

Figure 7.2 shows a plot of the vitamin C content of the tomatoes arranged according to variety (Fig. 7.2(a)–(c)) and as a single group (Fig. 7.2 (d)). The question of interest is whether the three varieties really produce tomatoes of different vitamin C content or whether the differences observed are simply random variation in samples drawn from the same population.

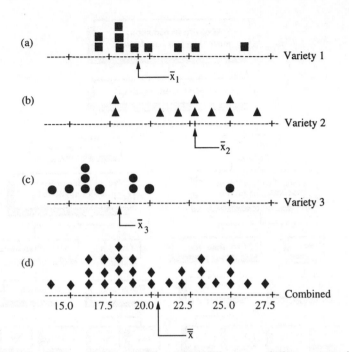

Fig. 7.2 Vitamin C content of tomatoes from three different varieties arranged (a), (b) and (c) according to variety and (d) as a combined group. $\bar{x}_1$, $\bar{x}_2$, $\bar{x}_3$ and $\bar{\bar{x}}$ are the mean vitamin C contents.

The basis of ANOVA is that if the three samples were really drawn from the same population (H_0: the three tomato varieties produce fruit with the same mean vitamin C content), then the within-varieties variance (σ_w^2) and the between-varieties variance (σ_b^2) are both estimates of the same population variance (σ^2).

In other words if H_0 were true, then the ratio σ_w^2/σ_b^2 should be approximately one. In practice one has to decide how far away from unity σ_w^2/σ_b^2 has to be before H_0 can be rejected. Therefore there is a need to know the probability distribution of σ_w^2/σ_b^2 or more precisely of s_w^2/s_b^2 where s_w^2 and s_b^2 are the sample variances. These are estimates of the true variances σ_w^2 and σ_b^2. Fisher showed that the ratio s_w^2/s_b^2 followed a distribution which was subsequently named in his honour as the F-distribution. There are many F-distributions (Fig. 7.3). If sample variances s_w^2 and s_b^2 are based on samples of sizes n_1 and n_2 from normal distributions $N(\mu_1, \sigma^2)$ and $N(\mu_2, \sigma^2)$ with the same variance σ^2, then the ratio s_w^2/s_b^2 follows the F-distribution with $(n_1 - 1)$ and $(n_2 - 1)$ degrees of freedom. The ratio s_w^2/s_b^2 is commonly referred to as the F-ratio.

Solution

To calculate the F-ratio, s_w^2 and s_b^2 are calculated first.

$$s_w^2 = \frac{1}{3}\left(s_1^2 + s_2^2 + s_3^2\right) \tag{7.1}$$

where s_1^2, s_2^2 and s_3^2 are the variances of samples from variety 1, variety 2 and variety 3 respectively. s_w^2 is simply $\frac{1}{3}$ of the sum of the three sample variances since under H_0, all three are samples from the same population.

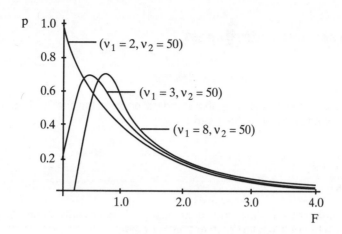

Fig. 7.3 *F*-distributions with different degrees of freedom (n_1 and n_2).

Calculating

$$s_1^2 = \frac{\sum_1^{10}(x_i - \bar{x}_1)^2}{(n_1 - 1)} \tag{7.2}$$

where $\bar{x}$ is the mean of vitamin C content of variety 1, x_i are the individual vitamin C contents of tomatoes from the variety, Σ is the summation symbol and n_1 is the sample size.

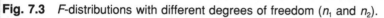

$$s_1^2 = \left[(26-19.8)^2 + (18-19.8)^2 + (22-19.8)^2 + (23-19.8)^2 + (17-19.8)^2 \right.$$
$$\left. + (18-19.8)^2 + (19-19.8)^2 + (17-19.8)^2 + (18-19.8)^2 + (20-19.8)^2\right]\big/(10-1)$$
$$= 26.766/9 = 8.844$$

Similarly

$$s_2^2 = \frac{\sum_1^{10}(x_i - \bar{x}_2)^2}{(n_2 - 1)}$$
$$= 8.711 \tag{7.3}$$

$$s_3^2 = \frac{\sum_1^{10}(x_i - \bar{x}_3)^2}{(n_3 - 1)}$$
$$= 10.233 \tag{7.4}$$

$$s_w^2 = \frac{1}{3}(8.844 + 8.711 + 10.233) = 9.263$$

$$s_b^2 = ns_{\bar{x}}^2$$

where n is the sample size and $s_{\bar{x}}^2$ is the standard error of the mean. This arises from the definition of the standard error of the mean.

Calculating

$$s_{\bar{x}}^2 = \frac{\sum\left(\bar{x}_i - \bar{\bar{x}}\right)^2}{k-1} \qquad (7.5)$$

where k is the number of samples; three in our case, $\bar{\bar{x}}$ is the overall mean and $\bar{x}_i$ is the mean of the ith variety where i takes values 1 to 3 in our case.

$$= \left[(19.8 - 20.033)^2 + (22.6 - 20.033)^2 + (17.7 - 20.033)^2\right] / (3-1)$$

$$= (12.087)/2 = 6.0433$$

$$s_b^2 = 10 \times 6.0433 = 60.433 \qquad \text{as the sample size is 10.}$$

$$F = s_b^2 / s_w^2$$
$$= 60.433/9.263 = 6.52 \qquad (7.6)$$

This is an F-value from the F-distribution with $(k-1)$ and $(1 + n_2 + n_3 - 3)$ or 2 and 27 degrees of freedom in the present case.

An F-value such as the one observed only occurs with a probability of about 0.005 under this F-distribution.

Figure 7.4 shows the F-distribution with 2 and 27 degrees of freedom. The critical value at a significance probability level of 0.05 and the observed F-value are also shown. The observed F-value is well within the critical region. H_0 is therefore rejected.

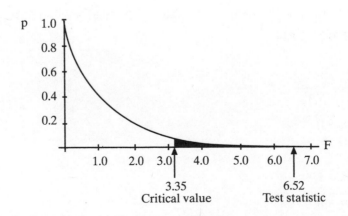

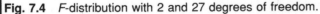

Fig. 7.4 F-distribution with 2 and 27 degrees of freedom.

Calculating the sum of squares given the variances

Note that the sum of squares within the samples which is also called the *error* or *residual sum of squares* (SSE) is given by

$$SSE = \sum_j \sum_i \left(x_{ji} - \bar{x}_j\right)^2 \tag{7.7}$$

$$SSE = \sum_{j=1}^{3} \sum_{i=1}^{10} \left(x_{ji} - \bar{x}_j\right)^2 \quad \text{in the present example} \tag{7.8}$$

$$SSE = \sum_{i=1}^{10} \left(x_i - \bar{x}_1\right)^2 + \sum_{i=1}^{10} \left(x_i - \bar{x}_2\right)^2 + \sum_{i=1}^{10} \left(x_i - \bar{x}_3\right)^2 \tag{7.9}$$

where j is the sample number and x_i is the observation within a given sample.

The between samples sum of squares which is also called the *explained* or *treatment sum of squares (SSTr)* is given by

$$SSTr = n \sum_{j=1}^{3} \left(\bar{x}_j - \bar{\bar{x}}\right)^2 \tag{7.10}$$

where n is the sample size and $\bar{x}_j$ the jth sample mean.

$$s_w^2 = SSR/(n_1 + n_2 + \ldots + n_k + k) \tag{7.11}$$

where k is the number of samples.

In the example

$$
\begin{aligned}
SSE &= (n_1 + n_2 + n_3 - 3)s_w^2 \\
&= (10 + 10 + 10 - 3)9.263 = 250.101
\end{aligned} \tag{7.12}
$$

$$s_b^2 \quad = SSTr/(k-1) \tag{7.13}$$

In our example

$$
\begin{aligned}
SSTr &= (k-1)s_b^2 \\
&= (3-1)60.433 = 120.866
\end{aligned} \tag{7.14}
$$

$$
\begin{aligned}
SSTo &= \sum_{i=1}^{30} \left(x_i - \bar{\bar{x}}\right)^2 \\
&= 370.97
\end{aligned} \tag{7.15}
$$

where i now takes values 1 to 30. SSTo can also be calculated from

$$
\begin{aligned}
SSTo &= SSE + SSTr \\
&= 250.101 + 120.866 = 370.97
\end{aligned}
$$

7.1.3 Tracing back

In illustrating the rationale underlying analysis of variance, the method was used to analyse results from a one factor experiment. The factor of concern was the variety of tomato. The response was the vitamin C content of the tomatoes expressed in mg per 100 g of fruit. The assumption made was that no other factors affected the response or if they did they affected each variety equally. This is achieved by growing the tomatoes under the same conditions. In other one-factor studies, such as in comparing the effectiveness of several treatments, the potential influence of other factors on the response is balanced out by assigning the experimental units to the treatments using an appropriate *randomisation* procedure (see Chapter 10). Tracing back the analysis of the data from the one-factor experiment, the following summary can be made.

7.1.4 Mechanics of one-way ANOVA

Step 1
Set up the null and alternative hypotheses.

H_0: the means are equal.
H_1: at least two of the means are unequal.

Step 2
Calculate the within-samples (or within-treatments) variance (s_w^2). This can be calculated from the within-samples or residual sum of squares (SSE) by dividing it by the degrees of freedom. $s_w^2 = \text{SSE}/(N - k)$ where N is the total number of experimental units and k is the number of independent samples.

Step 3
Calculate the between-samples (or between treatments) variance (s_b^2). This can be calculated from the between samples or treatments sum of squares (SSTr) by dividing it by the number of samples minus one.

$$s_b^2 = \text{STTr}/(k-1) \tag{7.13}$$

Step 4
Calculate the F-ratio = s_b^2/s_w^2. $\tag{7.6}$

Step 5
Compare the observed F-ratio with the critical value from the F-distribution with $(N - k)$ and $(k - 1)$ degrees of freedom.

Step 6
Draw conclusion.

7.1.5 *Analysis of variance table*

Very often the results of an ANOVA are presented in tabular form (as shown in Table 7.2) for a one-factor experiment. Applying this to our example on vitamin C content of tomatoes, using single precision arithmetic, the analysis of variance table for Example 7.1 is shown in Table 7.3.

Table 7.2 General layout for an ANOVA table.

Source	Degrees of freedom	Sum of squares	Mean sum of squares	F ratio
Factor	$(k-1)$	SSTr	$(SSTr)/(k-1)$	$(SSTr)/(N-k)$
Error	$(N-k)$	SSE	$(SSE)/(N-k)$	$(SSE)/(k-1)$
Total	$(N-1)$	SSTo		

Table 7.3 Analysis of variance table for data shown in Table 7.1.

Source	Degrees of freedom	Sum of squares	Mean sum of squares	F-ratio
Variety	2	120.87	60.43	6.52
Error	27	250.10	9.26	
Total	29	370.97		

7.1.6 *Computer solution*

Fortunately with computer packages such as MINITAB and SAS there is no need to calculate the different statistics long-hand. The output below shows how a one-way analysis of variance can be carried out by computer.

MINITAB format

One method of setting out the data for a one-way ANOVA in MINITAB is to enter the results for each variety of tomatoes in a separate column. The data in Table 7.4 show how the data are stored.

MINITAB commands

To perform the analysis one then simply issues the command

Table 7.4 MINITAB formatted data from Table 7.1.

Row	Variety		
	1	2	3
1	26	23	25
2	18	18	20
3	22	25	16
4	23	27	14
5	17	24	17
6	18	23	19
7	19	18	16
8	17	22	15
9	18	25	16
10	20	21	19

```
MTB > AOVoneway c1-c3
```

Objective

This tells MINITAB to carry out a one-way **A**nalysis **O**f **V**ariance on the data in columns 1 to 3.

MINITAB output

The results output by MINITAB are shown below:

```
ANALYSIS OF VARIANCE
SOURCE      DF        SS       MS       F        p
FACTOR       2    120.87    60.43    6.52    0.005
ERROR       27    250.10     9.26
TOTAL       29    370.97
                                    INDIVIDUAL 95 PCT CI'S FOR
                                    MEAN BASED ON POOLED STDEV
LEVEL        N      MEAN    STDEV    ------+------+------+---
Variety1    10    19.800    2.974         (-----*-----)
Variety2    10    22.600    2.951                    (---*---)
Variety3    10    17.700    3.199    (-----*-----)
                                    ------+------+------+---
POOLED STDEV =     3.044            17.5    20.0   22.5
```

Note:

- MINITAB also outputs the probability of observing the F-value indicated ($F = 6.52$) under H_0 as 0.005.
- MINITAB also gives the 95% confidence interval for the observed means based on the pooled variance. The pooled variance is calculated using the formula

$$s_p^2 = \frac{(n_1 - 1)s_1^2 + (n_2 - 1)s_2^2 + (n_3 - 1)s_3^2}{(n_1 + n_2 + n_3 - 3)}$$

$$= \frac{9 \times 2.974^2 + 9 \times 2.951^2 + 9 \times 3.199^2}{(10 + 10 + 10 - 3)}$$

$$= 3.044^2 \qquad\qquad (7.16)$$

The figures are obtained from the output given. Remember that variance is the square of the standard deviation.

The 95% confidence interval is calculated from

$$\bar{x}_i \pm t_{1-\alpha/2} s_{p/\sqrt{n_i}} = \bar{x}_i \pm t_{1-\alpha/2} \times \frac{3.044}{\sqrt{n_i}}$$

The t-value is from the t-distribution having the degrees of freedom associated with the s_w^2 term, 27 in our case.

For example, for sample 1 the 95% confidence interval is given by

$$\bar{x}_i \pm 2.052 \times 3.044/\sqrt{n_1}$$

or

$$19.8 \pm 2.052 \times 3.044/\sqrt{10} = [17.82,\ 21.77]$$

7.1.7 *Unequal sample sizes*

In the discussion so far it was assumed that the sample sizes were all equal to n and the appropriate analysis of variance table could be written as given in Table 7.5.

Table 7.5   Illustrating how the sum of squares is partitioned.

Source	DF	Sum of squares
Factor	$(k-1)$	$n\sum\limits_{j=1}^{k}\left(\bar{x}_j - \bar{\bar{x}}\right)^2$
Error	$(N-k)$	$\sum\limits_{j=1}^{k}\sum\limits_{i=1}^{n}\left(\bar{x}_{ji} - \bar{x}_j\right)^2$
Total	$(N-1)$	$\sum\limits_{j=1}^{k}\sum\limits_{i=1}^{n}\left(x_{ji} - \bar{\bar{x}}\right)^2$

Using equal sample sizes provides the most efficient design. However, this may not always be possible and some observations may be lost during the study. In such cases calculation of the treatment sum of squares is calculated using the formula

$$\sum_{j=1}^{k} n_j \left(\overline{x}_j - \overline{\overline{x}} \right)^2$$

Otherwise the calculations are essentially the same. However, estimation of variances may be biased.

7.1.8   *Assumptions about ANOVA and cautions*

One-way ANOVA assumes that:

- A random sample is drawn from each population.
- The populations have normal distributions with the same variance.

In practice, mild departures from normality do not cause too much problem. If the populations are markedly non-normal then the non-parametric Kruskal-Wallis method should be used. If sample sizes are not too different then mild departures from the equality of variances assumption can also be tolerated. On the other hand, biased samples may lead to totally erroneous conclusions.

7.2   Multiple range testing

In many experiments, we wish to compare more than two group means and very often investigators do this by examining each possible pair of groups separately using a test such as the Student's t-test (Chapter 5). With each of those tests our conclusion as to whether the two means being compared are the same or not is based on the probability of obtaining the observed difference, under the hypothesis of no difference.

A common end-point for rejection is an observed difference which is so large as to occur only 5% ($\alpha = 0.05$) of the time under the null hypothesis. As the number of such tests in the experiment increases the likelihood of detecting a significant difference when none actually exists, increases. In fact, the probability of finding at least one spurious significant result is given by $1 - (1 - \alpha)^n$ where α is the significance probability and n is the number of comparisons made. For example, for an experiment involving five groups and ten comparisons, the probability of detecting at least one significant result at an α level of 0.05 is $1 - (1 - 0.5)^{10}$ or 0.40 even though the group means are all from the same population.

To overcome this increased risk of finding a spurious significant result, analysis of variance is used. The null hypothesis being tested is, however, that all the group means are equal. A significant result, that is rejection of the null hypothesis, does not identify the pairs of means which are different. *Multiple range testing* does this while still controlling the overall (or experiment-wise) α level. Numerous methods are available including Scheffe's test, Tukey's test, Duncan's test and Newman-Keuls test (also called the Student Newman-Keuls test). Only the Tukey's test will be considered in this book because it is one of the simplest, has performed extremely well in simulation studies and allows calculation of a confidence interval for the estimate. References on the other methods are given at the end of this chapter.

7.2.1 *Procedure for Tukey's multiple-comparison test*

Step 1
Clarify question.
Make clear statement of problem.

Step 2
Formulate the null hypothesis.

$$H_0 : \mu_i = \mu_j \qquad \text{for any two treatment means.}$$

Step 3
Formulate the alternative hypothesis.

$$H_1 : \mu_i \neq \mu_j \qquad \text{for any two treatment means.}$$

Step 4
Calculate the test statistic.

$$\left| \bar{x}_i - \bar{x}_j \right| \bigg/ s\sqrt{\left[\left(1/n_i + 1/n_j\right)/2\right]} \tag{7.17}$$

Step 5
Compare the test value or statistic with critical value.

Critical value of the studentised range statistic $q(\alpha, k, v)$. This value is read from Tables just like any test statistic. Appendix 4 gives illustrative values.

Step 6
Decision: accept or reject the null hypothesis and reject or accept the alternative hypothesis.

Reject H_0 if test statistic $\geq$ critical value or equivalently

$|\bar{x}_i - \bar{x}_j| \geq q(\alpha, k, v)s\sqrt{[(1/n_i + 1/n_j)/2]}$ (called the honestly significant difference HSD)

where $\bar{x}_i$ and $\bar{x}_j$ are the estimates of μ_i and μ_j (the population means), s is the square root of the mean square error, n_i and n_j are the number of observations in groups i and j, α is the significance level, k is the number of treatment groups in the experiment, v is the degrees of freedom $(N - k)$ where $N = n_1 + n_2 + \ldots + n_k$ or the total number of observations in experiment and HSD is the honestly significant difference

$$= q(\alpha, \ k, \ v)s\sqrt{\left[(1/n_i + 1/n_j)/2\right]} \qquad \qquad (7.18)$$

Example 7.2

Suppose that in an experiment the mean responses are 591.6, 442.4, 348.4 and 290.8 units and the mean square error (s^2) is 3670 based on a 4×4 Latin square design.

Solution

$k = 4$, $N = 16$ with each group having 4 observations.

$$\text{HSD} = q(0.05, \ 4, \ 12)s\sqrt{\left[(1/n_i + 1/n_j)/2\right]}$$

$$= (4.20)\left(\sqrt{3670}\right)\left(\sqrt{\left[(1/4 + 1/4)/2\right]}\right) = 127.22$$

where the q value is obtained from Appendix 4.

$$|\bar{x}_1 - \bar{x}_2| = 591.6 - 442.4 = 149.20^*$$
$$|\bar{x}_1 - \bar{x}_3| = 591.6 - 348.4 = 243.20^*$$
$$|\bar{x}_1 - \bar{x}_4| = 591.6 - 290.8 = 300.80^*$$
$$|\bar{x}_2 - \bar{x}_3| = 442.4 - 348.4 = 94.00$$
$$|\bar{x}_2 - \bar{x}_4| = 442.4 - 290.8 = 151.60^*$$
$$|\bar{x}_3 - \bar{x}_4| = 348.4 - 290.8 = 57.60$$

where * denotes a significant difference.
These results can be summarised as follows:

1	2	3	4

Groups underlined by the same continuous line have the same mean response (e.g. there is no significant difference between the means of groups 2 and 3 in our test). Group means are arranged in decreasing numerical order from left to right (591.6, 442.4, 348.4 and 290.8 in Example 7.2).

7.3 Factorial ANOVA

In factorial ANOVA, the effect of more than one factor on a response variable is studied. Such investigations are discussed in Chapter 10.

7.4   Kruskal-Wallis test

The Kruskal-Wallis test is essentially a one-way analysis of variance using ranks. As the standard one-way ANOVA, it is used to determine whether k independent samples are from populations which differ in the characteristic of interest.

7.4.1   Rationale

Suppose that a number of samples are available and all the observations are ranked in a single series irrespective of which sample they came from. If the samples were from the same population or from populations with the same median then one would expect the average rank of the samples to be close to each other. On the other hand, if the samples came from populations with different medians, then the average ranks will be different.

7.4.2   Mechanics of the test

Step 1
Set up the null and alternative hypotheses.

Step 2
Rank the data as a single series. When ties are present give the ties the mean rank.

Step 3
Sum the ranks for each sample.

Step 4
Calculate the test statistic KW using the formula

$$KW = \frac{12}{N(N+1)} \sum_{j=1}^{k} \frac{R_j^2}{n_j} - 3(N+1) \tag{7.19}$$

where N is the total number of observations, n_j is the number of observations in the jth sample, R_j is the rank sum of the jth sample and k is the number of samples.

The test statistic is essentially the sum of squares deviation from the expected mean rank sum R but adjusted for different sample sizes and weighted for the effects of large samples.

If all the samples are of equal size n, then the test statistic becomes

$$KW = \frac{12}{n^2 k(nk+1)} \sum_{j=1}^{k} R_j^2 k - 3(nk+1) \tag{7.20}$$

The larger the KW value (remember the sum of squares deviation analogy), the stronger the evidence is against the null hypothesis that all rank sums are equal or that the population distributions are identical.

The null distribution of H converges to a χ^2_{m-1} distribution as the sample sizes increase.

Step 5
Compare the test statistic with the critical value (Neave, 1979).

Step 6
Make decision.

H_0 is rejected if KW $\geq$ critical value.

Example 7.3

In order to investigate the effect of biotin on the weight of premature babies, biotin was administered at a low (L) and high (H) dose by oral (O) or intravenous (I) administration. The four treatment combinations gave the following weight gains (g) after two weeks of therapy.

LO	250	252	197	199
LI	232	250	235	220
HO	255	241	239	240
HI	242	237	217	249

Parametric ANOVA is not suitable as the third and fourth baby in group LO show much smaller weight gains than the others. This suggests that variability in this group is wider than in the others thus violating one of the requirements for standard ANOVA.

Solution

Step 1
  H_0: The average weight gains in the four treatment groups are the same.
  H_1: The average weight gains are not all the same.

Step 2
Ranking the data.

LO	13.5	15	1	2
LI	4	13.5	5	3
HO	16	9	7	8
HI	10	6	11	12

Step 3
Rank sums.

$R_1 = 31.5$
$R_2 = 25.5$
$R_3 = 40$
$R_4 = 39$

Step 4
Test statistic

$$KW = \frac{12}{16 \times 4\left[(4 \times 4)+1\right]}\left\{31.5^2 + 25.5^2 + 40^2 + 39^2 - 3\left[(4 \times 4)+1\right]\right\}$$

$$= 1.53$$

Step 5
The critical region is ≥ 7.235 at a significance probability of 0.05 (Neave, 1979).

Step 6
Therefore H_0 of no treatment difference is accepted.

7.4.3   *Presence of many ties*

If there are many ties in the data, the variance of the sampling distribution of the test statistic KW will be markedly affected and a correction is recommended. This is done by dividing the KW value calculated earlier by

$$1 - \frac{\sum_{j=1}^{k}\left(t_j^3 - t_j\right)}{N^3 - N} \tag{7.21}$$

where k is the sample number, t_j is the number of tied ranks in the jth sample and N is the total number of observations across all the samples.

For example, if there were four samples with 2, 0, 4 and 1 ties respectively and the total number of observations were 40, then the correction factor is given by

$$\frac{1 - \left(2^3 - 2\right) + \left(0\right) + \left(4^3 - 4\right) + \left(1^3 - 1\right)}{40^2 - 40} = 0.979$$

This shows that unless there are many ties, the correction is negligible.

Chapter 8
Analysis of Covariance (ANCOVA)

8.1 Objectives

In many studies the objective is to investigate how a particular factor affects a response. Typically the means of two or more populations exposed to different levels of the factor of interest are compared, based on samples from each. In practice the populations may be entirely hypothetical. For example, when comparing treatments, subjects may be randomly allocated to the different treatment groups and their response measured after administration of the treatments. The responses of the groups are considered to be representative of the responses of hypothetical parent populations.

When subjects are randomly allocated to the different groups, the aim is to ensure that any differences in other factors, which may confound the results, are balanced out. This may not always be possible particularly with observational studies. For example, in a study comparing the mean vitamin E content of different varieties of a cereal, it may not be possible to harvest all the different varieties at the same stage of maturity. If it is known from previous experience that the more mature grains contain more vitamin E, then when analysing the data there is a need to *adjust* the results for differences in maturity. One of the most widely used methods for exercising such *statistical control*, when any of the measurable independent variables is not at predetermined levels, is analysis of covariance (ANCOVA).

Analysis of covariance is appropriate when the outcome factor is numerical, the treatment or risk factor is categorical and the confounding factor is numerical.

8.2 The general model and assumptions for ANCOVA

Suppose that the vitamin E (μg per 100 g) content of two varieties of barley can be represented by

$$Y_1 = \alpha_0 + \beta X + e \tag{8.1}$$

$$Y_2 = \alpha_1 + \beta X + e \tag{8.2}$$

where X is the maturity of the grain as measured by the fibre content and α_0 and α_1 are the expected vitamin E contents when $X = 0$. If the slopes β are the same in both equations then $(\alpha_1 - \alpha_0)$ represents the expected difference in vitamin E contents of the two barley varieties at the same stage of maturity x. This is shown graphically in Fig. 8.1.

Suppose that the two varieties are harvested at maturity levels x_1 and x_0 respectively. The expected vitamin E contents using equations Y_1 and Y_2 can therefore be represented as shown in Fig. 8.2.

In order to estimate the difference in mean vitamin E contents of the two varieties, one needs to adjust the observed values (y_1 and y_0) to y_{1a} and y_{0a}, the yields corresponding to the same maturity level x_a.

At maturity level x_a and x_1 the vitamin E contents of variety 1 are expected to be given by

$$y_{1a} = \alpha_1 + \beta x_a \qquad (8.3)$$

$$y_1 = \alpha_1 + \beta x_1 \qquad (8.4)$$

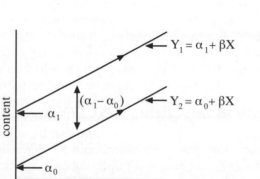

Fig. 8.1 Graph showing that the slopes of both lines are the same.

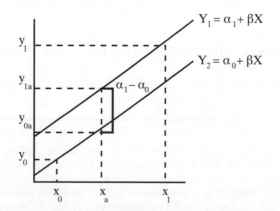

Fig. 8.2 Graph showing calculation of difference in intercepts.

so that

$$y_{1a} = y_1 - \beta(x_1 - x_a) \qquad (8.5)$$

Similarly

$$y_{0a} = y_0 - \beta(x_0 - x_a) \qquad (8.6)$$

Therefore

$$y_{1a} - y_{0a} = y_1 - y_0 - \beta(x_1 - x_0) \qquad (8.7)$$

To test whether there are real differences in vitamin E contents of the two varieties of barley one tests whether $\alpha_1 - \alpha_0 = 0$ or more commonly whether $\alpha_1 = \alpha_0$. The null hypothesis then takes the form

$$H_0 : \mu_0 = \mu_1$$

or more generally when there are n treatment groups

$$H_0 : \mu_0 = \mu_1 = \ldots = \mu_n$$

8.3 Assumptions underlying ANCOVA

The foregoing discussion underlines the assumptions of ANCOVA which are summarised here:

(1) There is a linear relationship between the response (Y) and the confounding variable (X).
(2) The slopes of the regression lines are the same for all treatment groups.
(3) The covariate is measured with no significant error.
(4) The error terms associated with the Y values are identically distributed independent normal variates. The normality assumption may however be relaxed.
(5) There are no unmeasured confounding variables.

Example 8.1

A study was carried out to compare two drugs claimed to reduce stress associated with the premenstrual syndrome. The degree of stress was evaluated by means of a questionnaire; the higher the score the more severe the degree of stress perceived by the patient. From previous experience those with more severe stress respond better than those who suffer less. Therefore, a pre-treatment score was measured for use as covariate. Table 8.1 gives the data.

Table 8.1 Pre- and post-treatment stress scores in patients treated with two drugs A and B.

Pre-score	Post-score	Drug code	Drug
11.0	9.8	A	1
10.1	10.2	A	1
13.1	10.7	A	1
14.0	10.9	A	1
14.4	11.2	A	1
15.4	11.3	A	1
16.1	11.7	A	1
17.7	11.8	A	1
18.1	12.2	A	1
19.0	12.3	A	1
18.8	12.9	B	0
11.0	10.7	B	0
12.0	10.8	B	0
13.2	11.1	B	0
13.5	11.6	B	0
15.0	11.7	B	0
16.2	11.6	B	0
17.0	12.8	B	0
16.3	12.5	B	0
18.3		B	0

Solution

To illustrate the procedures used to carry out an analysis of covariance (ANCOVA) by computer, the data in Table 8.1 were first read into a data file named ANCOVA2.dat. The pre-score data is given the variable name Prescore, the post-score data the name Postscor and the drug code used, the variable name Drug. MINITAB and SAS will be used to analyse the data.

SAS program

The SAS program to carry out the analysis of covariance is shown below:

Command	Objective
`Data ANCOVA1;`	Defines data file.
`Infile 'a:ANCOVA2.dat';`	Data retrieved from file.
	ANCOVA2.dat from disk a:
`Input Prescore Postscor Drug;`	Three columns read and given variable
`Run;`	names shown.
`PROC Print;`	Prints data input above.
`Run;`	
`PROC GLM;`	General linear model used.
`Class Drug;`	Drug is defined as qualitative variable.
`Model Postscor = Drug Prescore/`	Model defined with Prescore as covariate/
`Solution;`	coefficients printed.

```
Lsmeans drug/stderr;              Least squares mean response for each
                                    drug printed out with its standard error.
Output p = Predscor r = residual;  Predicted score and residual printed
PROC Print;                         out with labels shown.
Run;
```

SAS output 1

```
                    General Linear Models Procedure
                        Class Level Information

                  Class        Levels       Values

                  DRUG            2           0 1

                Number of observations in data set = 20

                    General Linear Models Procedure
```

Dependent Variable: POSTSCOR

		Sum of	Mean		
Source	DF	Squares	Square	F Value	Pr > F
Model	2	13.10699624	6.55349812	86.33	0.0001
Error	17	1.29050376	0.07591199		
Corrected Total	19	14.39750000			

R-Square	C.V.	Root MSE	POSTSCOR Mean
0.910366	2.390640	0.27552	11.5250000

Source	DF	Type I SS	Mean Square	F Value	Pr > F
DRUG	1	1.98450000	1.98450000	26.14	0.0001
PRESCORE	1	11.12249624	11.12249624	146.52	0.0001

Source	DF	Type III SS	Mean Square	F Value	Pr > F
DRUG	1	1.58056672	1.58056672	20.82	0.0003
PRESCORE	1	11.12249624	11.12249624	146.52	0.0001

Parameter	Estimate	T for H0: Parameter = 0	Pr > |T|	Std Error of Estimate
INTERCEPT	7.041408569 B	19.82	0.0001	0.35523480
DRUG 0	0.562809809 B	4.56	0.0003	0.12334184
1	0.000000000 B	.	.	.
PRESCORE	0.279959129	12.10	0.0001	0.02312856

Note: The X'X matrix has been found to be singular and a generalised inverse was used to solve the normal equations. Estimates followed by the letter 'B' are biased, and are not unique estimators of the parameters.

```
                    General Linear Models Procedure
                         Least Squares Means

           DRUG        POSTSCOR        Std Err          Pr > |T|
                        LSMEAN         LSMEAN       H0:LSMEAN = 0

            0        11.8064049      0.0871717            0.0001
            1        11.2435951      0.0871717            0.0001
```

OBS	PRESCORE	POSTSCOR	DRUG	PREDSCOR	RESIDUAL
1	11.0	9.8	1	10.1210	-0.32096
2	10.1	10.2	1	9.8690	0.33100
3	13.1	10.7	1	10.7089	-0.00887
4	14.0	10.9	1	10.9608	-0.06084
5	14.4	11.2	1	11.0728	0.12718
6	15.4	11.3	1	11.3528	-0.05278
7	16.1	11.7	1	11.5488	0.15125
8	17.7	11.8	1	11.9967	-0.19669
9	18.1	12.2	1	12.1087	0.09133
10	19.0	12.3	1	12.3606	-0.06063
11	18.8	12.9	0	12.8675	0.03255
12	11.0	10.7	0	10.6838	0.01623
13	12.0	10.8	0	10.9637	-0.16373
14	13.2	11.1	0	11.2997	-0.19968
15	13.5	11.6	0	11.3837	0.21633
16	15.0	11.7	0	11.8036	-0.10361
17	16.2	11.6	0	12.1396	-0.53956
18	17.0	12.7	0	12.3635	0.33648
19	16.3	12.8	0	12.1676	0.63245
20	18.3	12.5	0	12.7275	-0.22747

MINITAB program

In addition to the MINITAB ANCOVA command the REGRESS and the GLM commands will also be used for carrying out the analysis to further clarify the assumptions made in analysis of covariance.

MINITAB commands

ANCOVA command	Objective
MTB > ANCOVA 'Postscor' = 'DRUG';	Invokes the ANCOVA analysis and defines the model.
SUBC > covariate 'Prescore';	Defines the covariate.
SUBC > Fits C4;	The predicted values stored in C4.
SUBC > Resids C5;	The residuals stored in C5.
SUBC > Means Postscor.	The adjusted means printed.

MINITAB output 1

```
Factor      Levels      Values
Drug           2           0     1
```

```
Analysis of Covariance for PostScor

SOURCE          DF      ADJ SS          MS          F          p
Covariates      1      11.1225      11.1225      146.52      0.000
Drug            1       1.5806       1.5806       20.82      0.000
Error          17       1.2905       0.0759
Total          19      14.3975


Covariate       Coeff       Stdev      t-value                p
Prescore       0.2800      0.0231       12.10              0.000

ADJUSTED MEANS

Drug        N        PostScor
0          10         11.806
1          10         11.244

MTB > PRINT C1-C5

ROW       Prescore       PostScor       Drug        C4             C5

  1         11.0           9.8           1       10.1210       -0.320958
  2         10.1          10.2           1        9.8690        0.331005
  3         13.1          10.7           1       10.7089       -0.008872
  4         14.0          10.9           1       10.9608       -0.060836
  5         14.4          11.2           1       11.0728        0.127181
  6         15.4          11.3           1       11.3528       -0.052778
  7         16.1          11.7           1       11.5487        0.151250
  8         17.7          11.8           1       11.9967       -0.196684
  9         18.1          12.2           1       12.1087        0.091331
 10         19.0          12.3           1       12.3606       -0.060631
 11         18.8          12.9           0       12.8674        0.032551
 12         11.0          10.7           0       10.6838        0.016232
 13         12.0          10.8           0       10.9637       -0.163727
 14         13.2          11.1           0       11.2997       -0.199677
 15         13.5          11.6           0       11.3837        0.216334
 16         15.0          11.7           0       11.8036       -0.103604
 17         16.2          11.6           0       12.1396       -0.539556
 18         17.0          12.7           0       12.3635        0.336477
 19         16.3          12.8           0       12.1676        0.632449
 20         18.3          12.5           0       12.7275       -0.227469
```

MINITAB commands

Regress command

```
MTB > Regress 'Postscor'
  2 'Drug' 'Prescore'
```

Objective

Regression of Postscor data on 2 variables Drug and Prescor.

MINITAB output 2

```
The regression equation is
Postscor = 7.60 - 0.563 drug + 0.280 Prescore
```

Predictor	Coef	Stdev	t-ratio	p
Constant	7.6042	0.3606	21.09	0.000
drug	-0.5628	0.1233	-4.56	0.000
Prescore	0.27996	0.02313	12.10	0.000

```
s = 0.2755      R-sq = 91.0%      R-sq(adj) = 90.0%
```

Analysis of Variance

SOURCE	DF	SS	MS	F	p
Regression	2	13.1070	6.5535	86.33	0.000
Error	17	1.2905	0.0759		
Total	19	14.3975			

SOURCE	DF	SEQ SS
drug	1	1.9845
Prescore	1	11.1225

Unusual Observations

Obs.	drug	Postscor	Fit	Stdev.Fit	Residual	St.Resid
17	0.00	11.6000	12.1396	0.0906	-0.5396	-2.07R
19	0.00	12.8000	12.1676	0.0912	0.6324	2.43R

```
R denotes an obs. with a large st. resid.
```

MINITAB commands

The analysis can also be carried out using the MINITAB GLM command.

GLM command	Objective
`MTB > GLM Postscor = drug;`	Defines model and invokes the general linear model approach.
`SUBC > Covariate Prescore.`	Defines the covariate.

MINITAB output 3

Factor	Levels	Values	
Drug	2	0	1

Analysis of Variance for PostScor

Source	DF	Seq SS	Adj SS	Adj MS	F	p
Prescore	1	11.5264	11.1225	11.1225	146.52	0.000
drug	1	1.5806	1.5806	1.5806	20.82	0.000
Error	17	1.2905	1.2905	0.0759		
Total	19	14.3975				

```
Term            Coeff        Stdev       t-value              p
Constant       7.3228       0.3526        20.77          0.000
Prescore       0.27996      0.02313       12.10          0.000

Unusual observations for Postscor

Obs.      Postscor         Fit     Stdev. Fit      Residual     St. Resid
17        11.6000     12.1396        0.0906       -0.5396         -2.07R
19        12.8000     12.1676        0.0912        0.6324          2.43
```

R denotes an obs. with a large st. resid.

Interpretation

To understand the SAS and MINITAB ANCOVA outputs, first consider the MINITAB regression output (MINITAB output 2). The model used was

$$\text{Postscor} = \alpha + \beta_1(\text{Drug}) + \beta_2(\text{Prescore}) + \varepsilon \tag{8.8}$$

and from the output the regression line was given by the following equation

$$\text{Postscor} = 7.60 - 0.563 \text{ Drug} + 0.280 \text{ Prescore} \qquad \text{SSReg} = 13.1070.$$

Also given is the regression sum of square. If the regression is now repeated twice ignoring the variable Drug and Prescore respectively the following regression equations are obtained

$$\text{Postscore} = 7.25 + 0.285 \text{ [Prescore]} \qquad \text{SSReg} = 11.526 \tag{8.9}$$

$$\text{Postscore} = 11.8 - 0.630 \text{ [Drug]} \qquad \text{SSReg} = 1.9845 \tag{8.10}$$

The sum of squares due to the two variables are therefore given by

$$\text{SS(Drug)} = 13.1070 - 11.526 = 1.581$$
$$\text{SS(Prescore)} = 13.1070 - 1.9845 = 11.1225$$

These sums of squares are listed as the adjusted sum of squares (Adj SS) in the MINITAB ANCOVA output and as the type III SS in the SAS output. The appropriate *F*-values are then calculated from the mean square and the mean square error (MSE). The latter is obtained from the full model including both Drug and Prescore as variables.

$$F\text{-value (Drug)} = \frac{1.581/1}{0.0759} \approx 20.83$$

$$F\text{-value (Prescore)} = \frac{11.1225/1}{0.0759} \approx 146.54$$

Using the full precision of the SAS outputs the *F*-values are 20.82 and 146.52 as listed.

The adjusted means

The mean prescore values for subjects receiving drug A and B are 15.13 and 14.89 respectively. The overall mean prescore is therefore equal to 15.01. The prediction equation is given by

Postscore = 7.604 − 0.563 [Drug] + 0.280 [Prescore]   (8.11)

Therefore for drug A the *adjusted* mean score is

Postscore = 7.604 − 0.563 [1] + 0.280 [15.01] = 11.244

and for drug B

Postscore = 7.604 − 0.563 [0] + 0.280 [15.01] = 11.807

Hence, the adjusted mean difference is (11.80 − 11.24) = 0.563. This is of course also the difference between the intercepts as ANCOVA assumes that the lines are parallel. In this case the adjusted mean postscore is not much different to the unadjusted means (11.84 − 11.21) = 0.63. From the SAS output the p value for $H_0 : \beta_1 = 0$ is 0.0003. The MINITAB output shows that p is <0.001. There is, therefore, a difference in response to drugs A and B.

8.4   Checking the validity of ANCOVA

To test the assumption that the linear regression lines are parallel one can either test for the slopes or intercepts being equal.

This is easily done by SAS or MINITAB. A third variable, produced by multiplying the variables Prescore and Drug, is created to give the model

$$\text{Postscore} = \alpha + \beta_1[\text{Drug}] + \beta_2[\text{Prescore}] + \beta_3[\text{Drug} \times \text{Prescore}] + \varepsilon \quad (8.12)$$

For drug A therefore

$$\text{Postcore} = \alpha + \beta_1 + (\beta_2 + \beta_3)[\text{Prescore}] + \varepsilon \quad (8.13)$$

and for drug B

$$\text{Postscore} = \alpha + \beta_2[\text{Prescore}] + \varepsilon$$

Therefore β_3 gives the difference in slopes between the two regression lines. The null hypothesis for no difference in slopes is $H_0 : \beta_3 = 0$. Running the regression analysis, β_3 is estimated to be −0.019 with a p value of 0.689. Therefore, the estimate is consistent with a mean difference in slope of zero. Hence there is insufficient evidence to reject the null hypothesis that the two lines are parallel.

8.5   Caution

In addition to ensuring that the assumptions made in ANCOVA (parallelism and linearity) are met, the values of the covariable should also show considerable overlap for the treatment groups. Otherwise, extrapolation beyond the ranges applicable for the different groups may be required. Such extrapolation carries a high risk of producing erroneous estimates.

In Example 8.1 illustrated, ANCOVA was applied to data from a study in which the subjects were randomly assigned to the different treatments. Such a design is called a completely randomised design (see Chapter 10). There were also no missing data. Such a design is *orthogonal*. More generally, an orthogonal design is one which enables the total sum of squares to be uniquely partitioned into distinct additive (or orthogonal) components. While the GLM command can handle missing data, the MINITAB ANCOVA command requires orthogonal designs and eliminates any row containing missing data. This means that orthogonal designs, such as the latin square and cross-over designs, cannot be analysed by the ANCOVA design if there are missing data. In such cases and with non-orthogonal designs such as the incomplete block design, the GLM command should be used. Fortunately MINITAB warns of the danger by printing out the warning, 'Unequal cell counts'.

Chapter 9
Analysis of Categorical Data

9.1 Objective

In this chapter statistical methods commonly used for the analysis of categorical data are described (see also Fig. 9.1) and cautions in their use highlighted. Correlation analysis of categorical data is discussed in Chapter 6.

9.2 Chi-square test

The chi-square (χ^2) test is used to test whether a set of data fits a given statistical model or to test whether there are associations between variables.

9.2.1 Background

- Is there an association between type of housing and incidence of colds in occupants?
- Is it true that women are bad drivers?
- Is it true that individuals of the same educational background but in different jobs show different affinities to share ownership?
- Is it true that dental caries occur with different frequencies in different ethnic groups?

To answer such questions a test for association is required between the variables. The chi-square test is one test for association between categorical variables as well as ordinal variables. The chi-square test also enables testing for goodness of fit to a specific statistical model (e.g. Poisson distribution) or to a specific biological or scientific model (e.g. Mendel's second law).

Arranging the data so that one variable (e.g. colour of eyes) is along one axis and a second (e.g. severity of reaction to sunlight) is along the other axis, forms a two-way *contingency table*. A third variable (e.g. gender) can be superimposed on one of the axes to form a more complicated three-way contingency table. In this discussion only two-way contingency tables will be considered. In contingency tables the data are given in counts not percentages.

9.2.2 Mechanics of the test

Step 1
Set up a contingency table with the observed (O) values.

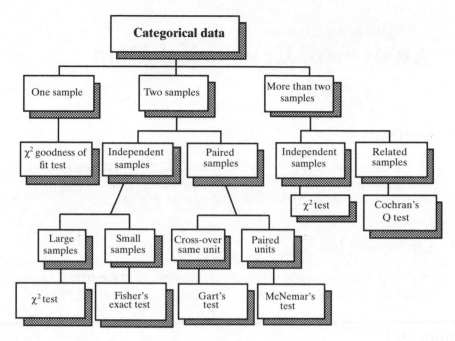

Fig. 9.1   Flow diagram for analysis of categorical data.

Step 2
Set up the null and alternative hypothesis.

Step 3
Calculate the expected frequencies for each cell (E).

Step 4
Calculate the chi-square statistic, χ^2

$$\chi^2 = \sum \frac{(O-E)^2}{E}$$ (9.1)

Each term in the sum refers to a specific cell.

Step 5
Compare the test statistic with the critical value obtained from the chi-square distribution with ν degrees of freedom (see also Fig. 9.2).

$$\nu = (r-1)(c-1)$$ (9.2)

where r is the number of categories for variable 1 (rows) and c is the number of categories for variable 2 (columns).

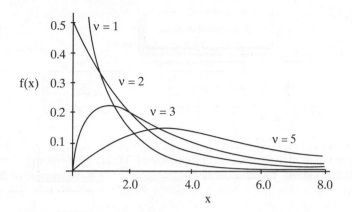

Fig. 9.2 χ_n^2 distribution for degrees of freedom ν.

The χ^2 statistic is a sum of residuals related term. There the critical, or rejection of null hypothesis, region consists of values larger than the critical value (Appendix 5).

Example 9.1

An experiment was carried out to test whether the response to sunlight was different in individuals with different eye colours. 100 individuals were recruited and classified according to eye colour. Each individual was then exposed to a minimal erythemal dose (MED) of ultraviolet light (UV). This dose was determined using a set of brown-eyed volunteers. The reactions shown by the 100 subjects four hours after receiving the MED of UV light are summarised in Table 9.1. Use the χ^2 test to determine whether the colour of eyes affected the response.

Table 9.1 Dermal response of individuals exposed to a given dose of ultra violet light shown to be the average erythemal dose in a group of brown-eyed individuals.

Eye colour	Sunlight reaction			Total
	Peeling	Erythema	No reaction	
Observed values:				
blue	25	28	6	59
green	5	5	7	17
brown	6	10	15	31
Total	36	43	28	107
Expected values:				
blue	59 × 36/100 = 19.85	23.71	15.44	59
green	5.72	6.83	4.45	17
brown	10.43	12.46	8.11	31
Total	36	43	28	107

Solution

$$\chi^2 \text{ statistic} = \sum \frac{(\text{observed value} - \text{expected value})^2}{\text{expected value}}$$

$$= \frac{(25 - 19.85)^2}{19.85} + \frac{(28 - 23.71)^2}{23.71} + \ldots + \frac{(15 - 8.11)^2}{8.11}$$

$$= 18.14 \tag{9.3}$$

This is a value from the χ^2 distribution with $(3 - 1)(3 - 1) = 4$ degrees of freedom.

The critical value at a significance probability of 0.05 is 11.14 and 14.86 at $\alpha = 0.01$ (see Appendix 5 and Neave, 1979).

Therefore, the data provide strong evidence that people with different eye colours react differently to the same dose of ultraviolet radiation.

9.2.3   Yates' continuity correction for the 2 × 2 table

When deriving the distribution for the statistic χ^2, the chi-square distribution, which is a *continuous* probability distribution, is used to approximate a discrete probability distribution (count data in the contingency table). Yates (1934) suggested that the approximation is improved if 0.5 is subtracted from each positive discrepancy between the observed value and the expected value and 0.5 is added to each negative discrepancy. The formula for calculating the χ^2 statistic then becomes

$$\chi^2 = \sum \frac{(|O - E| - 0.5)^2}{E} \tag{9.4}$$

where $|O - E|$ means the absolute value or modulus, ignoring sign.

There is no consensus as to whether such a correction is indeed useful. Introducing the correction produces a smaller χ^2 value. Therefore the rejection rule is more conservative with the uncorrected χ^2 value than with the corrected value. Therefore, whether the corrected or uncorrected value is used can be referred to how important the consequences of rejection of the null hypothesis are. In general, use of the corrected value is recommended particularly with the smaller sample sizes.

9.2.4   Chi-square goodness-of-fit model

The chi-square distribution may be used to determine whether observations fit particular probability models.

Example 9.2

In studying the cross-fertilisation of peas, Mendel produced his now famous second law of the inheritance of genes. Table 9.2 gives a set of data from one of his experiments and the values predicted by his theory. Using the data given carry out a hypothesis test that the law is valid.

Table 9.2 Mendel's data on cross-fertilised peas.

	Round/Yellow	Round/Green	Wrinkled/Yellow	Wrinkled/Green	Total
			Characteristic		
Observed	315	108	101	32	556
Expected	312.7	104.3	104.3	34.7	556

Solution

The χ^2 statistic is given by

$$\chi^2 = \sum \frac{(O_i - E_i)^2}{E_i}$$

$$= \frac{(315 - 312.7)^2}{312.7} + \frac{(108 - 104.3)^2}{104.3} + \frac{(101 - 104.3)^2}{104.3} + \frac{(32 - 34.7)^2}{34.7}$$

$$= 0.463$$

The critical χ^2 value at $\alpha = 0.05$ level and 3 degrees of freedom is 9.348 (see Appendix 5).

There is therefore no good evidence to reject H_0 that Mendel's law is obeyed.

9.2.5 χ^2 dispersion test

One form of the chi-square test is useful for testing whether occurrences in space are random. This is essentially a goodness-of-fit test.

Example 9.3

Suppose that in a study of cases of a new disease, a large rural area where the population is even was divided into 16 equal quadrats and the number of affected people was counted in each quadrat with the following results:

10, 9, 8, 12, 16, 11, 5, 14, 16, 10, 11, 12, 13, 14, 15, 16.

Is there any evidence for clustering of cases?

Solution

If the pattern is random (H_0) then it can be shown that the statistic $[(k-1)s^2]/\bar{x}$ follows a chi-square distribution with $(k-1)$ degrees of freedom where k is the number of quadrats, s^2 the sample variance and $\bar{x}$ is the sample mean.

$$\frac{(k-1)s^2}{\bar{x}} \qquad \text{can be rewritten as} \qquad \sum \frac{(O_i - E_i)^2}{E_i}$$

If the cases occur randomly in space

E_i = mean number of cases per quadrat

$$= (10 + 9 + 8 + \ldots + 16)/16$$

$$= 12.$$

The test statistic

$$\chi^2 = \frac{(10-12)^2}{12} + \frac{(9-12)^2}{12} + \ldots + \frac{(16-12)^2}{12} = 12.5$$

The critical value at α = 0.05 level is 27.488 (see Appendix 5 for the χ^2 distribution with 15 degrees of freedom). There is therefore no good evidence against the null hypothesis that the cases of the new disease occur randomly in space.

9.3   Fisher's exact test

When the sample sizes in the 2×2 contingency table being analysed are small (at least one cell with fewer than five counts), the χ^2 approximation to the distribution of the χ^2 statistic can be very poor. In such cases *Fisher's exact test* should be used. For fixed marginal totals (see Table 9.3) and *two independent variables*, the distribution is that associated with sampling without replacement from a finite population and is known as the *hypergeometric distribution*.

Table 9.3   Contingency table showing marginal totals.

		Variable 1		Marginal totals
		Category A	Category B	
Variable 2	Category A	a	b	$a + b$
	Category B	c	d	$c + d$
Marginal totals		$a + c$	$b + d$	

Example 9.4

In a study comparing two drugs in two groups of similar patients, the incidence of gastric ulceration was monitored by endoscopy and the data shown in Table 9.4. Is there sufficient evidence to conclude that one drug is less likely to induce the adverse effect?

Solution

Step 1

Given contingency table – Table 9.4.

Table 9.4 Contingency table for Example 9.4.

		Drug A	Drug B	Total
Adverse effect	Yes	2	5	7
	No	20	17	37
Total		22	22	44

Step 2

$H_0 : P_A = P_B$ i.e. proportion with adverse effects in the two groups are identical.

$H_1 : P_A < P_B$ Drug A is less likely to cause the adverse effect than, drug B.

Step 3

$$P_A = \frac{(a+b)!\,(c+d)!\,(a+c)!\,(b+d)!}{a!\,b!\,c!\,d!\,N!}$$

$$= \frac{7!\,37!\,22!\,22!}{2!\,5!\,20!\,22!\,44!} = 0.1587438$$

Step 4

More extreme outcomes than that given in the contingency table shown by Table 9.4 are shown in Table 9.5.

Table 9.5 Two extreme outcomes for Example 9.4.

		Drug A	Drug B	Total			Drug A	Drug B	Total
Adverse effect	Yes	1	6	7	Adverse effect	Yes	0	7	7
	No	21	16	37		No	22	15	37
Total		22	22	44	Total		22	22	44

9.3.1 *Mechanics of the test*

Step 1

Set up the (2 × 2) contingency table.

Step 2

Set up the null and alternative hypothesis.

Step 3

Calculate the probability of the observed outcome using the formula

$$p_A = \frac{(a+b)!\,(c+d)!\,(a+c)!\,(b+d)!}{a!\,b!\,c!\,d!\,N!} \qquad (9.5)$$

where a, b, c and d are the entries in the 2×2 contingency table as shown in Table 9.3. (!) is the factorial sign and N the total number of experimental units studied, i.e. $(a + b + c + d)$.

Step 4
Calculate the probabilities associated with outcomes more extreme than that observed, namely

$$p_{a-1},\ p_{a-2},\ \ldots,\ p_0$$

Step 5
The probability of obtaining the observed distribution shown in the contingency table and more extreme outcomes is given by

$$p = p_a + p_{a-1} + p_{a-2} + \ldots + p_0 \qquad (9.6)$$

Step 6
Reject H_0 if p is smaller than the critical p required (e.g. 0.05 at the 5% level); otherwise accept H_0.

The probabilities associated with those outcomes are

$$p_1 = \frac{7!\,37!\,22!\,22!}{1!\,6!\,21!\,16!\,44!} = 0.0428356$$

$$p_0 = \frac{7!\,37!\,22!\,22!}{0!\,7!\,22!\,15!\,44!} = 0.0044505$$

Note that 0! is defined as 1.

So, continuing the case in Example 9.4, the rest of the solution is:

Step 5
$p = p_0 + p_1 + p_2 = 0.2060299 \simeq 0.206$

Step 6
At the 0.05 level, H_0 cannot be rejected.

9.3.2   *Points to note*

- The χ^2 test is a two-tailed test whereas Fisher's exact test is a one-tailed test. The direction of departure from the null hypothesis in Fisher's exact test depends on the observed data. Remember that Fisher's statistic is calculated from the probability of obtaining the observed distribution of counts under H_0 plus the probabilities associated with more extreme arrangements, *in the same direction* as the observed arrangement.
- Large sample sizes are required to detect even moderately large differences between two proportions using Fisher's exact test. Therefore, while Fisher's

exact test is particularly useful when sample sizes are small it must be remembered that the risk of accepting H_0 when it is untrue is usually high.

9.4 McNemar's test

The chi-square test and Fisher's exact test assume that the samples are independent. When the samples are made up of matched pairs, as is often the design in many studies (e.g. matching of subjects according to sex, severity of disease or age), alternative tests are required. One such test is *McNemar's test*.

9.4.1 *Mechanics of the test*

Step 1
Set up a contingency table with the observed (O) values.

Step 2
Set up the null and alternative hypotheses.

Table 9.6 Contingency table for the McNemar test.

Characteristic		Sample 1		Total
		Absent	Present	
Sample 2	Present	a	b	$a + b$
	Absent	c	d	$c + d$
Total		$a + c$	$b + d$	$a + b + c + d$

Step 3
Calculate the McNemar statistic (the test statistic). Given the contingency table shown in Table 9.6, the McNemar statistic (also given the symbol χ^2) is given by

$$\chi^2 = \frac{(|a - d| - 1)^2}{a + d} \tag{9.7}$$

or

$$\chi^2 = \frac{(a - d)^2}{a + d} \tag{9.8}$$

Step 4
Compare the test statistic with the critical value obtained from the χ^2 distribution with 1 degree of freedom.

Example 9.5

In an experiment comparing the ability of two cell culture media (A and B) to grow the HIV virus, 60 blood samples from infected individuals were each incubated in the two cultures with the results shown below:

Sample

(1)	growing in both media A and B	25
(2)	growing in media A but not B	5
(3)	growing in media B but not A	16
(4)	failing to grow in both A and B	14
	Total	60

Do the data provide sufficient evidence to claim that the media are different in their suitability for growing the viruses?

Solution

Step 1

The data can be presented as a contingency table – see Table 9.7.

Table 9.7   Contingency table for Example 9.5.

		Cell culture A		Total
		No growth	Growth	
Cell culture B	Growth	16	25	41
	No growth	14	5	19
Total		30	30	60

Step 2

$H_0 : p_A = p_B$ equal proportion of specimens showing growth in the two media.
$H_1 : p_A \neq p_B$

Step 3

McNemar statistic

$$\chi^2 = \frac{(|a - d| - 1)^2}{a + d} = \frac{(|16 - 5| - 1)^2}{21} = 4.76$$

Step 4

The critical χ^2 value at 0.05 level with 1 degree of freedom is 3.84 (see Appendix 5). Since the test statistic is 4.76 there is strong evidence that medium B is better than A for growing the virus.

Q9.1

In a study to investigate whether a debate on vaccination affects the uptake of vaccination of infants by parents, 75 parents were asked whether they wished to vaccinate their children against whooping cough (pertussis) before and after watching a television debate on the subject. The following results were recorded:

No. of parents
Approving vaccination both before and after debate	27
Approving vaccination before but not after debate	13
Approving vaccination after but not before debate	7
Disapproving vaccination both before and after debate	28

Did watching the debate have any influence on uptake of vaccination?

A9.1

Step 1
The contingency table can be written as shown in Table 9.8.

Table 9.8 Contingency table for Question Q9.1.

		Before debate		Total
		Disapprove	Approve	
After debate	Approve	7	27	34
	Disapprove	28	13	41
Total		35	40	75

Step 2

$H_0 : p_a = p_b$ i.e. equal proportion of interviewees disapprove of vaccination both before and after watching the debate.

$H_1 : p_a \neq p_b$ proportions of interviewees disapproving the debate are not equal.

Step 3
McNemar statistic

$$\chi^2 = \frac{\left(|7 - 13| - 1\right)^2}{20} = 1.25$$

Step 4
Critical value for χ^2 distribution at 0.05 level and 1 degree of freedom is 3.84 (see Appendix 5). Therefore there is insufficient evidence to show that watching the debate actually influenced the parents' views about pertussis vaccination.

9.5 Gart's test

In some study designs, observations are paired in such a way that there are possible period or sequence effects. A typical example arises when a group of subjects are given a particular treatment on one occasion and then crossed-over to receive a second treatment. A particular response (e.g. incidence of side-effects) is noted during both occasions to determine whether there are any differences between the two treatments. Period or sequence effects therefore need to be accounted for. *Gart's test* does this.

9.5.1 Mechanics of the test

Step 1
Set up contingency table for the test as shown in Table 9.9.

Table 9.9 Contingency table for Gart's test.

	Treatment order (A, B)	(B, A)	Total
Response with A	a	b	$a + b$
Response with B	c	d	$c + d$
Total	$a + c$	$b + d$	$a + b + c + d$

Step 2
Set up the null hypothesis and the alternative hypothesis.

Step 3
Perform a Fisher's exact test on the data as laid out in step 1.

Step 4
Make decision; reject H_0 if the observed p is smaller than the critical p (0.05 at the usual 5% level).

Example 9.6
In a study of whether the order in which two drugs (A and B) are given affects the incidence of coughing induced by them, the data shown in Table 9.10 were collected. What conclusions can be drawn from the data?

Table 9.10 Patients developing cough during drug treatments A and B.

		Drug order (A, B)	(B, A)	Total
Cough	Present with A	4	2	6
	Present with B	7	3	10
Total		11	5	16

Solution

Step 1
Already given in Table 9.6.

Step 2
$H_0 : p_1 = p_2$ i.e. order of drug administration has no effect.
$H_1 : p_1 \neq p_2$ i.e. order of administration affects the outcome.

Step 3
Applying Fisher's exact test $p = 0.654$.

Step 4
H_0 cannot be rejected; order of administration does not appear to affect the outcome.

Note that the data can be used to test for treatment differences by reorganising the contingency table as Table 9.11.

Table 9.11 Reorganising Table 9.10.

		Drug order (A, B)	(B, A)	Total
Adverse effect	First drug	4	3	7
	Second drug	7	2	9
Total		11	5	16

Applying Fisher's exact test $p = 0.365$.
Again there is insufficient evidence to indicate real treatment differences with respect to cough induction.

Chapter 10
Further Experimental Design

10.1 Objective

In the discussion so far experimental data have been considered alongside observational data without precisely defining the differences between those two types of studies. The distinction is made clear in this chapter. The types of experiments considered in earlier chapters are summarised and more complicated designs introduced (see Fig. 10.1). The use of multiple linear regression for the analysis of experimental data is illustrated. The analysis of data from observational studies are considered in Chapter 11.

10.2 What are experiments?

The term experiment has several meanings. Most applied scientists take the term to mean any study in which data are collected to gain further insight into a scientific phenomenon. From a statistical standpoint the term experiment refers to any study in which at least one response is measured as a function of one or more variables which are set at specific levels by the experimenter.

What separates an experiment from an observational study is that in the former the investigator has control over the independent variable(s) or treatment administered whereas in the latter this is not the case. In many experiments the objective is to compare the effect of several treatments on a response. Such experiments are sometimes referred to as critical, or comparative, experiments.

10.3 What is experimental design?

In every experiment the investigator attempts to evaluate how specific factors (the treatment) affect a measurable outcome (the response). For example, the aim may be to evaluate the effect of heat on product yield. To quantitatively ascribe any change in the yield to temperature it is necessary to ensure that any other factors (e.g. presence of catalytic impurities or pressure) which may affect it do not vary, or alternatively vary to the same extent, during the different experimental runs at different temperatures. If several factors which affect the response alter simultaneously during the experiments and data is available only on one of the factors (e.g.

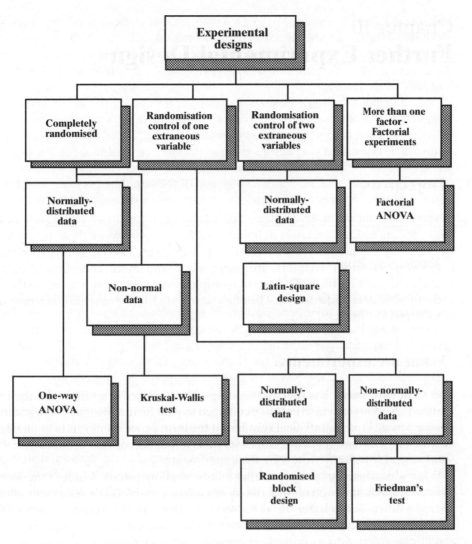

Fig. 10.1 Some commonly used experimental designs and their associated hypothesis tests.

temperature), then it is not possible to dissociate the effect of that factor from those of the other factors. In such cases the other factors are said to be *confounding variables*, in that they make quantitative assignment of effects to the factor of interest impossible, and the estimate of any effect observed is said to be *biased*.

Experimental design refers to the overall plan of an experiment to ensure that estimates of effects of treatments are unbiased. The term *treatment* is used here in a very general sense to describe any agent or procedure which is applied specifically to affect the response under investigation. It may therefore, for example, be a drug, a specific animal feed, a particular patient-education method or a particular microbial culture medium. The *plan* would include definition of the precise hypotheses to be tested, the selection of experimental units on which observations of the response are to be made, the assignment of the experimental units to the treatment groups, the definition of the experimental conditions and the methods of analysis of the results.

When defining the hypotheses to be tested and selecting the experimental units and the treatments to be used, the experimental designer must bear in mind whether the aim is to obtain a true measure of the effect of the treatment on the individuals concerned (i.e. ensure *internal validity*) or to obtain results which can be applied to a wider group or population (i.e. *external validity*). To achieve the latter often requires an in-depth knowledge of the scientific problem being investigated. For this reason, the discussion of experimental design will largely centre on ensuring internal validity.

10.4   Reducing bias

The prime objective of experimental design is to reduce and hopefully, eliminate bias in the estimates of effects. Two broad approaches are used, often concurrently for controlling bias. The *first* approach attempts to reduce bias by ensuring that the groups or experimental units being compared are as alike as possible with respect to confounding *factors*. When the confounding factors cannot be identified, the only approach to reduce bias is by the *second* approach, *randomisation* or by the use of the same experimental unit as its own. In practice both approaches are used. With randomisation an experimental unit has an equal probability to any other of being assigned to any of the treatment groups. Use of the same unit as its own control (a within-subjects design), although intuitively attractive introduces a potential problem, namely the introduction of time sequence in the administration of the treatments as a possible confounding factor particularly when the treatments have long-lasting effects which carry over (*carry-over effects*) into the periods when a different treatment is being administered. This is discussed further under cross-over and repeated measures designs.

10.5   The completely randomised design (CRD)

The CRD can be regarded as a generalisation of the two independent samples design. Instead of randomly assigning the experimental units or subjects to receive one of two treatments, the assignments are made to a number of different groups. Typically, therefore, the completely randomised design is used when one wishes to compare the effect of several treatments on a response variable. Indeed, analysis of data arising from a study using such a design has already been discussed in Chapter 7 under single factor analysis of variance (one-way ANOVA) and the Kruskal-Wallis test. Therefore aspects of the CRD design discussed there will not be repeated here.

10.6   Randomisation procedures

Randomisation does not mean haphazard. Randomisation procedures which reduce the risk of biased sample selection are necessary to ensure reliable estimates of the true effects of treatments. One, of the most common procedures for randomisation uses a table of random numbers (e.g. Appendix 11 or computer generated).

To illustrate how this is done, consider an experiment in which three treatments are to be compared. Suppose that 18 subjects are to be randomly allocated to the three treatments. The following random numbers were generated using the MINITAB commands:

```
MTB > Random      50     C1
MTB > INTEGER      0      9
MTB > PRINT              C1


4    8    1    1    9    9    2    7    7    9    3    2    1    8    7
3    6    7    2    2    1    8    3    0    4    3    2    0    7    1
3    4    4    4    2    0    8    5    1    0    8    3    3    8    8
2    4    9    8    3
```

Any table of random numbers could have been used instead. The assignment rule is that numbers 0, 1 and 2 will be assigned to treatment 1; 3, 4 and 5 to treatment 2 and 6, 7 and 8 to treatment 3. Number 9 will be discarded. Aligning the random numbers against the subject number produces the following sequence.

Subject	1	2	3	4	5	6	7	8	9	10	11	12	13	14	15	16	17	18
Random number	4	8	1	1	2	7	7	3	2	1	8	7	3	6	2	3	4	3
Treatment	2	3	1	1	1	3	3	2	1	1	3	3	2	3	1	2	2	2

Note that once a treatment has six subjects allocated, all subsequent random numbers which assign subjects to that treatment are ignored. Such random numbers are identified in **bold** in the list above. When there are more that ten treatments, double digits (neighbouring random numbers) may be used to allocate random numbers to the treatments and so on.

The last three assignments to treatment 2 could have been done without reference to the random numbers since only that treatment has an insufficient number of subjects at those stages.

10.7   Randomised block experiments

Sometimes it may not be possible to obtain experimental units which are sufficiently homogeneous for an experiment with a completely randomised design to be useful. Such a situation arises when, for example, the effects of several fertilisers are to be compared and it is necessary to use more than one field each of which show different fertilities. Each field may then be considered as a block which is subdivided into plots. If it is possible to block (e.g. fields) the experimental units (e.g. plots) in such a way that within block variability, with respect to some possible confounding variable (e.g. fertility), is smaller than between block variability, then the design would be more sensitive than the completely randomised design. It is, however, important that blocking is used only when there is clear evidence of heterogeneity which can be blocked out. In addition to blocking out variation, the randomised block design provides a wider inductive basis than an experiment carried out with uniform experimental units. In other words, the treatments are tested on units with different characteristics and the conclusions drawn apply to this wider group too.

10.7.1 The model

$$y_{ij} = \mu + \tau_i + \beta_j + e_{ij} \tag{10.1}$$

where y_{ij} is the response of the experimental unit in the jth block receiving ith treatment, μ is a constant, τ_i is the treatment effect, β_j is the block effect and e_{ij} is the error term $E \sim N(0, \sigma^2)$.

$$SSTo \quad = \quad SSTr \quad + \quad BSS \quad + \quad SSE$$

Where SSTo is the total sum of squares, SSTr is the explained sum of squares or treatment sum of squares, BSS is the block sum of squares and SSE is the residual or error sum of squares.

10.7.2 The ANOVA table for a randomised block experiment

To separate treatment and block effects from random variation, the sum of squares are partitioned as shown in Table 10.1.

Table 10.1 Partitioning sum of squares.

Source of variation	Degrees of freedom	Sum of squares	Mean square	F-value
Treatments	$k-1$	SSTr	$MSTr = SSTr/(k-1)$	MSTr/MSE
Blocks	$l-1$	BSS	$MSB = BSS/(l-1)$	
Error	$(k-1)(l-1)$	SSE	$MSE = SSE/((k-1)(l-1))$	
Total	$(kl-1)$	SSTo		

10.7.3   Blocking

The classical example of blocking is an experiment designed to evaluate the effect of different varieties of a crop on yield. Blocking is used to overcome problems associated with being unable to have plots which are sufficiently homogeneous. Each block is chosen so that plots within it have more homogeneity, with respect to soil fertility and other factors affecting growth, than plots over the whole experimental area.

Some further examples of blocking are:

(1)   Evaluation of analytical methods using each operator or technician as a block or alternatively evaluating the performance of technicians using a series of equipments as blocks.
(2)   Comparing different formulations of a given vaccine using each animal or a subject as a block.
(3)   Comparing different fermentation processes for the production of an antibiotic with different blends of the mother liquor acting as blocks.
(4)   Comparing different packaging on sales of a product using blocks consisting of retail outlets which are as similar as possible, e.g. supermarkets with a given turnover and corner shops.
(5)   Comparing different training schemes on the performance of children using social backgrounds as a basis for blocking.
(6)   Comparing growth-promoting effects of a series of different diets in mice using litters as blocks.

Assumptions that are made when using randomised block experiments are:

● Any single observation made on any particular treatment in a given block is assumed to be from a normal distribution.
● The variance is the same for each block–treatment combination.

10.7.4   Typical arrangement for a randomised block experiment

The treatments for a randomised block experiment, such as that described at the start of Section 10.7.3, may be randomly allocated to each block as shown in Table 10.2. Note that the treatments (T1, T2 and T3) within each block are randomised.

Table 10.2   Treatment allocations in different blocks.

Block 1	Block 2	Block 3	Block 4
T2	T2	T1	T1
T1	T1	T2	T3
T3	T3	T3	T2

10.7.5   The sum of squares

The sum of squares are defined as:

Treatment $$\mathrm{SSTr} = b \sum_{i=1}^{k} \left(\bar{y}_{i\bullet} - \bar{y}_{\bullet\bullet} \right)^2$$ (10.2)

Block $$\mathrm{BSS} = k \sum_{j=1}^{b} \left(\bar{y}_{\bullet j} - \bar{y}_{\bullet\bullet} \right)^2$$ (10.3)

Residual $$\mathrm{SSE} = \sum_{i=1}^{k} \sum_{j=1}^{b} \left[\bar{y}_{ij} - \left(\bar{y}_{i\bullet} - \bar{y}_{\bullet\bullet} \right) - \left(\bar{y}_{\bullet j} - \bar{y}_{\bullet\bullet} \right) - \bar{y}_{\bullet\bullet} \right]^2$$ (10.4)

Total $$\mathrm{SSTo} = \sum_{i=1}^{k} \sum_{j=1}^{b} \left(\bar{y}_{\bullet j} - \bar{y}_{\bullet\bullet} \right)^2$$ (10.5)

sum over b blocks.
sum over k treatments.

where $y_{i\bullet}$ is the ith treatment mean,
$\bar{y}_{\bullet j}$ is the jth block mean,
y_{ij} is the observation from the jth block with the ith treatment and

$$y_{ij} = \bar{y}_{\bullet\bullet} + \left(\bar{y}_{i\bullet} - \bar{y}_{\bullet\bullet} \right) + \left(\bar{y}_{\bullet j} - \bar{y}_{\bullet\bullet} \right) + \left(\bar{y}_{\bullet j} - \bar{y}_{i\bullet} - \bar{y}_{\bullet j} + \bar{y}_{\bullet\bullet} \right)$$ (10.6)

The dot subscripts indicate which averages are being considered. For example, the double dotted average refers to the average value over both blocks and treatment.

10.7.6   The analysis

Consider the data shown in Table 10.3. The sum of squares may be calculated using the equations given in Section 10.7.5.

Table 10.3   Data from a randomised block experiment.

	Crop yields (kg) in different plots arranged in blocks after three treatments				Treatment mean
	Block 1	Block 2	Block 3	Block 4	
Treatment 1	75.000	70.000	85.000	92.000	80.500
Treatment 2	84.000	78.000	94.000	92.000	87.000
Treatment 3	80.000	72.000	83.000	85.000	80.000
Block mean	79.667	73.333	87.333	89.667	82.500

$$3\sum_{j=1}^{4}\left(\bar{y}_{\bullet j}-\bar{y}_{\bullet\bullet}\right)^2 = \begin{bmatrix} 79.667\ 73.333\ 87.333\ 89.667 \\ 79.667\ 73.333\ 87.333\ 89.667 \\ 79.667\ 73.333\ 87.333\ 89.667 \end{bmatrix} - \begin{bmatrix} 82.5\ 82.5\ 82.5\ 82.5 \\ 82.5\ 82.5\ 82.5\ 82.5 \\ 82.5\ 82.5\ 82.5\ 82.5 \end{bmatrix}$$

$$= \begin{bmatrix} -2.833\ -9.167\ 4.833\ 7.167 \\ -2.833\ -9.167\ 4.833\ 7.167 \\ -2.833\ -9.167\ 4.833\ 7.167 \end{bmatrix} \rightarrow \text{sum squared} \begin{array}{l} = \text{BSS} \\ = 500.33 \end{array}$$

$$4\sum_{i=1}^{3}\left(\bar{y}_{i\bullet}-\bar{y}_{\bullet\bullet}\right)^2 = \begin{bmatrix} 80.5\ 80.5\ 80.5\ 80.5 \\ 87.0\ 87.0\ 87.0\ 87.0 \\ 80.0\ 80.0\ 80.0\ 80.0 \end{bmatrix} - \begin{bmatrix} 82.5\ 82.5\ 82.5\ 82.5 \\ 82.5\ 82.5\ 82.5\ 82.5 \\ 82.5\ 82.5\ 82.5\ 82.5 \end{bmatrix}$$

$$= \begin{bmatrix} -2 & -2 & -2 & -2 \\ 4.5 & 4.5 & 4.5 & 4.5 \\ -2.5 & -2.5 & -2.5 & -2.5 \end{bmatrix} \rightarrow \text{sum squared} = \text{SSTr} = 122.00$$

$$\sum_{i=1}^{k}\sum_{j=1}^{b}\left(\bar{y}_{ij}-\bar{y}_{\bullet\bullet}\right)^2 = \begin{bmatrix} 75\ 70\ 85\ 92 \\ 84\ 78\ 94\ 92 \\ 80\ 72\ 83\ 85 \end{bmatrix} - \begin{bmatrix} 82.5\ 82.5\ 82.5\ 82.5 \\ 82.5\ 82.5\ 82.5\ 82.5 \\ 82.5\ 82.5\ 82.5\ 82.5 \end{bmatrix}$$

$$= \begin{bmatrix} -7.5 & -12.5 & -2.5\ 9.5 \\ 1.5 & -4.5 & -11.5\ 9.5 \\ -2.5 & -10.5 & 0.5\ 2.5 \end{bmatrix} \rightarrow \text{sum squared} = \text{SSTo} = 677$$

$$\text{SSTo} = \text{SSTr} + \text{BSS} + \text{SSE}$$

10.7.7   The ANOVA table

The ANOVA table for the data given in Table 10.3 may be seen in Table 10.4.
    The value in adopting a complete *block* randomised design instead of a completely randomised design can be seen by comparing the ANOVA tables for the two designs using data from Tables 10.4 and 10.5.

Table 10.4   ANOVA table for the data given in Table 10.3.

Source of variation	Degrees of freedom	Sum of squares	Mean square	F statistic
Treatment	2	122.00	61.00	6.7
Block	3	500.33	166.78	
Error	6	54.67	9.11	
Total	11	677.00		

Table 10.5   ANOVA table for the data given in Table 10.3 ignoring blocks.

Source of variation	Degrees of freedom	Sum of squares	Mean square	F statistic
Treatment	2	122.0	61.0	0.99
Error	9	555.0	61.7	
Total	11	677.0		

The ANOVA table for the completely randomised design is shown in Table 10.5.

10.7.8   The conclusion

The critical F-value for the hypothesis test with 2 and 6 degrees of freedom at a significance probability of 0.05 is 5.14 (Appendix 3).

The test statistic from Table 10.4 is greater than the critical value. Hence, the null hypothesis is rejected and the alternative hypothesis that at least two of the means are different is accepted.

If the data are analysed ignoring the blocks, the critical F-value with 2 and 9 degrees of freedom is 4.26. Since the test statistic is 0.99 (Table 10.5), the null hypothesis cannot be rejected.

Blocking has, therefore, enabled the detection of differences which were masked by inter-block variability. Indeed, blocking reduced the residual or error sum of squares to about 10% of the original value. Note, however, that blocking leads to a reduction in degrees of freedom and should therefore only be resorted to when there is clear evidence of heterogeneity in the blocks.

10.8   Friedman's test

This involves distribution-free analysis of data from randomised block experiments.

The Friedman's test is based on evaluating a residual sum of squares adjusted with a multiplier to obtain a distribution which tends towards the χ^2 distribution with $m-1$ degrees of freedom as sample size tends to infinity. Therefore the larger the value of Friedman's test statistic (M) the smaller the significance probability will be.

The test is essentially a distribution-free two-way analysis of variance. However, Friedman's test, unlike parametric analysis of variance, does not allow estimation of treatment difference through the use of contrasts. The emphasis is therefore on hypothesis testing. Sample sizes must be equal to the number of blocks for each treatment.

The test statistic is:

$$M = \frac{12}{am(m+1)} \sum_{k=1}^{m} R_k^2 - 3a(m+1)$$ (10.7)

where m is the number of blocks, a is the number of treatments and R_k is the rank sum for the kth treatment.

10.8.1   *Mechanics of the Friedman's test*

Step 1
Arrange data into relevant blocks and treatments.

Step 2
Rank the results in each block with the lowest required change ranked 1.

Step 3
Calculate Friedman's test statistic (M).

Step 4
Look up the critical value at the significance probability required (Neave, 1979). If M is greater than the critical value then the null hypothesis: that there are no treatment differences, is rejected.

Example 10.1

An experiment was carried out to determine whether calcium and oestrogens were effective in a group of hospitalised patients suffering from post-menopausal osteoporosis. All the patients included in the study were screened to be as homogeneous in disease severity and physiological

Table 10.6   Effect of various diets on bone density.

Block	Treatment		
	Control diet	Control diet + 3 g calcium daily	Control diet + 2 × 1.25 mg conjugated oestrogens daily
1	1.0	1.0	1.1
2	0.8	0.9	1.1
3	0.7	1.0	1.2
4	0.9	1.1	1.3
5	1.0	0.9	1.2
6	1.1	1.2	1.6
7	1.2	1.3	0.9
8	0.9	1.4	1.0
9	0.9	0.9	1.7
10	0.8	0.9	1.6

indices as possible. This was easier using blocks of three patients because of patient heterogeneity. The effect of treatment on bone density was assessed by X-ray analysis using a new image analysis technique on the resultant negative film. The output is in terms of an opacity ratio ranging from 0 (no density detectable) through 1 (no improvement) to 2 (improvement to normal opacity ratio). The results obtained after 3 months' treatment were as shown in Table 10.6.

Solution

Step 1
The data are arranged as in Table 10.6.

Step 2
Ranking the data according to improvement gives Table 10.7.

Step 3
Calculating Friedman's test statistic

$$= \frac{12}{30(3+1)}\left(26^2 + 21^2 + 13^2\right) - 3 \times 10(3+1) = 8.6$$

Step 4
Critical value at a significance probability of 0.05 is 6.2 (Neave, 1979).

There is strong evidence that the treatments produce different results. The oestrogens are more effective than the other two treatments.

Table 10.7   Ranking the data given in Table 10.6.

Block	Treatment		
	Control diet	Control diet + 3 g calcium daily	Control diet + 2 × 1.25 mg conjugated oestrogens daily
1	2*	2*	1
2	3	2	1
3	3	2	1
4	3	2	1
5	2	3	1
6	3	2	1
7	1	2	3
8	3	1	2
9	2*	2*	1
10	3	2	1
Rank sum	26	21	13

*Equal ranks.

10.9   The Latin square design

The Latin square design can be regarded as blocking in two directions. In agricultural trials, for example, fertility trends may exist along both the length and width of a large field. By blocking along both directions, the variability due to them may be eliminated and identification of main effects are therefore made easier.

10.9.1   Features of the Latin square design

Table 10.8 shows the features of Latin square designs:

(1)   The number of levels for each of the two variables used to block the experimental units is equal to the number of treatments. For example, in Table 10.8 there are five levels of each of factor A and factor B.
(2)   Each level of each factor occurs only once along each row and each column.

Table 10.8   A 5 × 5 Latin square design.

Levels		Factor I			
	1	2	3	4	5
1	A	B	C	D	E
2	B	C	D	E	A
Factor II 3	C	D	E	A	B
4	D	E	A	B	C
5	E	A	B	C	D

10.9.2   Some applications of the Latin square design

In their investigation of the sedative effects of a anti-allergic drug (meclastine), Hedges *et al.* (1971) used a placebo (dummy tablet) and a second drug (promethazine) for comparison. They used a 3 × 3 Latin square design with day of study and volunteer as the block systems. They replicated the Latin square three times thereby using nine volunteers in total.

In a study by Al-sereiti *et al.* (1989), three eye-drop formulations were compared for their pressure lowering effects. The authors used a double-blind, cross-over and balanced design based on 3 × 3 Latin squares. Intra-ocular pressure was the response variable and the formulation was the treatment. The subjects and the occasion on which the drop was studied were the blocking variables. Nine subjects were recruited for the three Latin squares.

10.10 Advantages and disadvantages of specific experimental designs

The relative advantages and disadvantages of the completely randomised, the randomised block and the Latin square designs are summarised in Table 10.9.

Table 10.9 Advantages and disadvantages of completely randomised, randomised block and Latin square experimental designs.

		Design				
		Completely randomised		Randomised block		Latin square
Advantages	(1) (2) (3)	Easy to conduct. Easy to analyse even with unequal samples sizes. Can be used for any number of treatments.	(1) (2)	Efficient method for controlling the effect of an extraneous source of variability. Can accommodate a large number of treatments.	(1)	Efficient way of controlling the effects of two extraneous variables.
Disadvantages	(1)	The experimental units have to be as homogeneous as possible.	(1) (2) (3)	The number of treatments which can be accommodated is limited since the experimental units have to be homogeneous within each block. Only one extraneous variable is controlled. Each treatment effect must be approximately the same from block to block.	(1) (2)	The number of treatments which can be accommodated is usually small. Each treatment effect must be approximately the same across both extraneous treatment variables.

10.11 Factorial designs

A factorial experiment is one in which the effects of more than one factor are investigated simultaneously in all their possible combinations.

The simplest factorial experiment involves two factors each set at two levels. Such an experiment may, for example, be one in which the effects of two factors

Table 10.10 The layout for a 2×2 factorial experiment.

Experimental run	pH	Ionic strength
1	Low	Low
2	Low	High
3	High	Low
4	High	High

(pH and ionic strength) on product yield (the response) in an enzymic reaction, is studied at two levels (arbitrarily labelled high and low). There will, therefore, be four experimental runs as shown in Table 10.10.

10.11.1 Terminology

A factorial design such as the one just described is referred to as a 2×2 or 2^2 factorial experiment. Similarly, an experiment involving three factors each at two levels is referred to as a 2^3 factorial experiment. Generally, factorial experiments in which n factors are each set at two levels are called 2^n factorial experiments. Likewise, 3^n experiments are those involving n factors each fixed at three levels. Factorial experiments may also have the factors set at different levels. For example, a $2 \times 3 \times 5$ factorial experiment is one with three factors at two, three and five levels respectively.

10.11.2 Why use factorial experiments?

Factorial experiments offer several advantages over other commonly used experimental design:

(1) Factorial experiments are more efficient than those in which each factor is altered in turn while the others are held constant. For example, consider an experiment in which the effect of two factors on a response is to be studied. A commonly used design is as shown in Table 10.11.

Suppose that in such an experiment, $4n$ experimental units are used. If the factorial design shown in Table 10.12 is used, only $2n$ experimental units are required for the same precision in the estimates of the effects of factors A and B.

(2) Factorial designs enable effects of one factor to be estimated at more than one level of the other factors thereby improving the *generalisability* of the results. In other words the conclusions hold for a wider range of conditions.

(3) Factorial designs enable the investigation of interaction between different factors and hence help to avoid erroneous conclusions.

Consider the results of a 2×2 factorial experiment shown in Table 10.12 and Fig. 10.2.

Table 10.11 A commonly used design for studying the effect of changing levels of two factors.

Experimental run	Level A	Level B	Number of experimental units
1	Low	Constant	n
2	High	Constant	n
3	Constant	Low	n
4	Constant	High	n

Table 10.12 Results of 2×2 factorial design.

		Factor B	
		L (low)	H (high)
Factor A	L (low)	10	20
	H (high)	40	10

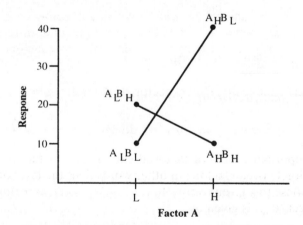

Fig. 10.2 Results of a 2×2 factorial design.

The results show clearly that the response to A depends on the levels of factor B. If a one-at-a-time design was used and the factor B level was held at low then the conclusion would have been that increasing factor A increases the response from 10 to 40. If now factor A is maintained constant and factor B altered from low to high, an increased response from 10 to 20 is observed. It would, therefore, be tempting to conclude that increasing the levels of both A and B to H would produce an even higher response. From Fig. 10.2, it can be seen that that conclusion would have been erroneous because of the A and B interaction.

10.11.3   Effects in a factorial experiment

Several effects can be measured in a factorial experiment. Firstly, let the mean responses to the different treatments shown in Fig. 10.2 be represented as follows:

μ_{10} = mean response to treatment $A_H B_L$
μ_{00} = mean response to treatment $A_L B_L$
μ_{01} = mean response to treatment $A_L B_H$
μ_{11} = mean response to treatment $A_H B_H$

The effect (μ_{A0}) of factor A when B is held at level L is therefore given by

$$\mu_{A0} = \mu_{10} - \mu_{00} \tag{10.8}$$

and the effect (μ_{A1}) of factor A when B is held at level H is given by

$$\mu_{A1} = \mu_{11} - \mu_{01} \tag{10.9}$$

The *main effect* of factor A (θ_A) is defined as the mean response ($\mu_{A0} + \mu_{A1}$)/2 that is,

$$\theta_A = 0.5\left[\left(\mu_{10} - \mu_{00}\right) + \left(\mu_{11} - \mu_{01}\right)\right] \tag{10.10}$$

Similarly, the *main effect* of factor B (θ_B) is given by

$$\theta_B = 0.5\left[\left(\mu_{01} - \mu_{00}\right) + \left(\mu_{11} - \mu_{10}\right)\right] \tag{10.11}$$

An important aspect of factorial experiments is the investigation of possible interaction between factors; in other words does the level of another factor affect the response to a given factor? In the 2×2 factorial experiment the mean interaction effect (θ_{AB}) is given by

$$\theta_A = 0.5\left[\left(\mu_{11} - \mu_{01}\right) - \left(\mu_{10} - \mu_{00}\right)\right] \tag{10.12}$$

An alternative notation which is commonly used in textbooks uses μ_1, μ_a, μ_b and μ_{ab} to represent μ_{00}, μ_{10}, μ_{01} and μ_{11} respectively. Therefore the main and interaction effects can be represented by

$$\theta_A = 0.5\left[\left(\mu_a - \mu_1\right) + \left(\mu_{ab} - \mu_b\right)\right] \tag{10.13}$$

$$\theta_B = 0.5\left[\left(\mu_b - \mu_1\right) + \left(\mu_{ab} - \mu_a\right)\right] \tag{10.14}$$

$$\theta_{AB} = 0.5\left[\left(\mu_{ab} - \mu_b\right) - \left(\mu_a - \mu_1\right)\right] \tag{10.15}$$

Note: The interaction effect is really given by the difference between the effects of factor A when factor B is high and low, that is,

$$0.5\left[\left(\mu_{11} - \mu_{10}\right) - \left(\mu_{10} - \mu_{00}\right)\right] \qquad \text{or} \qquad 0.5\left[\left(\mu_{ab} - \mu_{b}\right) - \left(\mu_{a} - \mu_{1}\right)\right]$$

but is defined as half of this as (θ_{AB}) because by so doing the variance is the same as those of the main effects θ_A and θ_B.

10.11.4 Variance of estimated effects

Suppose that in the 2×2 factorial experiment considered, each treatment group $(A_L B_L, A_L B_H, A_H B_L$ and $A_H B_H)$ had n subjects or experimental units in each. In other words the experiment is *balanced*. If the true variance of the data is σ^2 then one would expect each treatment group to have this variance too. Therefore the *mean* response of each group is expected to be σ^2/n.

Now, the main effect of factor A is given by

$$\theta_A = 0.5\left[\mu_a - \mu_b + \mu_{ab} - \mu_b\right] \tag{10.16}$$

with each of the μ values having a variance of σ^2/n. Therefore the variance of θ_A is given by

$$V\left(\theta_A\right) = \frac{1}{4}\left[\frac{\sigma^2}{10} + \frac{\sigma^2}{10} + \frac{\sigma^2}{10} + \frac{\sigma^2}{10}\right] = \frac{\sigma^2}{10} \tag{10.17}$$

since the variance of $ah(x)$ where a is a constant and $h(x)$ is a function of x (e.g. $x_1 + x_2 + x_3 + x_4$) is given by $V(ah(x)) = a^2 \, V(h(x)) = a^2 \, V(x_1 + x_2 + x_3 + x_4)$ where x_1, x_2, x_3 and x_4 are *independent* random variables. The true variance σ^2 is estimated by the pooled variance s^2 given by

$$s^2 = \frac{\left(n-1\right)s_1^2 + \left(n-1\right)s_2^2 + \left(n-1\right)s_3^2 + \left(n-1\right)s_4^2}{\left(n_1-1\right)\left(n_2-1\right)\left(n_3-1\right)\left(n_4-1\right)} \tag{10.18}$$

The estimated variance of $\hat{\theta}_A$, the estimate of θ_A is therefore given by

$$V\left(\hat{\theta}_A\right) = \frac{s^2}{10} \tag{10.19}$$

$s^2/10$ is an estimate of the variance of $\hat{\theta}_B$ and $\hat{\theta}_{AB}$, the estimates of θ_B and θ_{AB} as defined above.

A pooled variance is used because an assumption of the F-test is that the samples are independent and drawn from populations with the same variance.

10.12   Analysing data from designed experiments using multiple regression and the generalised linear model by computer

10.12.1   Randomised block design

To illustrate how the linear model for the randomised block design is expressed as a linear equation relating the response, Y, to a series of class variables, X, representing the different blocks and treatments, consider the experiment shown in Table 10.13.

Seven different class variables, X, can be chosen to represent the three blocks and four treatments so that the responses can be written as follows:

$$Y = \alpha + \tau_1(X1) + \tau_2(X2) + \tau_3(X3) + \tau_4(X4) + \beta_1(X5) + \beta_2(X6) + \beta_3(X7) + \varepsilon$$

The individual responses can therefore be expressed as:

$$y_{11} = \alpha + \tau_1(1) + \tau_2(0) + \tau_3(0) + \tau_4(0) + \beta_1(1) + \beta_2(0) + \beta_3(0) + \varepsilon_{11}$$
$$y_{12} = \alpha + \tau_1(0) + \tau_2(1) + \tau_3(0) + \tau_4(0) + \beta_1(1) + \beta_2(0) + \beta_3(0) + \varepsilon_{12}$$
$$y_{13} = \alpha + \tau_1(0) + \tau_2(0) + \tau_3(1) + \tau_4(0) + \beta_1(1) + \beta_2(0) + \beta_3(0) + \varepsilon_{13}$$
$$y_{14} = \alpha + \tau_1(0) + \tau_2(0) + \tau_3(0) + \tau_4(1) + \beta_1(1) + \beta_2(0) + \beta_3(0) + \varepsilon_{14}$$
$$y_{21} = \alpha + \tau_1(1) + \tau_2(0) + \tau_3(0) + \tau_4(0) + \beta_1(0) + \beta_2(1) + \beta_3(0) + \varepsilon_{21}$$
$$y_{22} = \alpha + \tau_1(0) + \tau_2(1) + \tau_3(0) + \tau_4(0) + \beta_1(0) + \beta_2(1) + \beta_3(0) + \varepsilon_{22}$$
$$y_{23} = \alpha + \tau_1(0) + \tau_2(0) + \tau_3(1) + \tau_4(0) + \beta_1(0) + \beta_2(1) + \beta_3(0) + \varepsilon_{23}$$
$$y_{24} = \alpha + \tau_1(0) + \tau_2(0) + \tau_3(0) + \tau_4(1) + \beta_1(0) + \beta_2(1) + \beta_3(0) + \varepsilon_{24}$$
$$y_{31} = \alpha + \tau_1(1) + \tau_2(0) + \tau_3(0) + \tau_4(0) + \beta_1(0) + \beta_2(0) + \beta_3(1) + \varepsilon_{31}$$
$$y_{32} = \alpha + \tau_1(0) + \tau_2(1) + \tau_3(0) + \tau_4(0) + \beta_1(0) + \beta_2(0) + \beta_3(1) + \varepsilon_{32}$$
$$y_{33} = \alpha + \tau_1(0) + \tau_2(0) + \tau_3(1) + \tau_4(0) + \beta_1(0) + \beta_2(0) + \beta_3(1) + \varepsilon_{33}$$
$$y_{34} = \alpha + \tau_1(0) + \tau_2(0) + \tau_3(0) + \tau_4(1) + \beta_1(0) + \beta_2(0) + \beta_3(1) + \varepsilon_{34}$$

One of the difficulties when solving a system of equations such as that shown, is that some of the columns are linearly dependent. For example, the coefficients of the first column can be obtained by a linear combination of the coefficients of columns 2 to 5 or of columns 6 to 8. The X matrix is said to be not of *full rank*

Table 10.13 Arrangement of y observations from a randomised block experiment with three blocks and four treatments each.

Block	Treatment			
	1	2	3	4
1	y_{11}	y_{12}	y_{13}	y_{14}
2	y_{21}	y_{22}	y_{23}	y_{24}
3	y_{31}	y_{32}	y_{33}	y_{34}

because of *singularities*. In other words, these are too many parameters (α_1, τ_1, τ_2, τ_3, τ_4, β_1, β_2 and β_3) to be estimated and these have to be reduced in number. This is done by imposing constraints on some of the parameters. This is called reparameterisation to make the matrix full rank. One of the commonest types of constraints imposed on such equations is called the corner constraint. This is done by setting τ_1 and β_1 equal to zero. The responses can therefore be rewritten such that all the terms including τ_1 and β_1 are set at zero.

To illustrate the practical application of the approach just described, suppose that the twelve y values observed were as shown:

y_{11}	y_{12}	y_{13}	y_{14}	y_{21}	y_{22}	y_{23}	y_{24}	y_{31}	y_{32}	y_{33}	y_{34}
4.4	3.3	4.4	6.8	5.9	1.9	4.0	6.5	6.1	5.0	4.6	6.9

MINITAB or SAS can be used to fit the data to the model

$$Y = \alpha + \tau_2(X2) + \tau_3(X3) + \tau_4(X4) + \beta_2(X6) + \beta_3(X7) + \varepsilon \tag{10.20}$$

The data matrix is as shown in Table 10.14.

MINITAB commands

Objective

MTB > Regress C1 5 C2-C6   The response *y* is regressed against the three class variables (*X2*, *X3* and *X4*) representing treatments 2, 3 and 4 and the two class variables (*X6*, *X7*) representing blocks 2 and 3.

Table 10.14   Indicator values for various observations.

	Column					Treatment	Block
C1	C2	C3	C4	C5	C6		
		Variable					
Y1	X2	X3	X4	X6	X7		
4.4	0	0	0	0	0	1	1
3.3	1	0	0	0	0	2	1
4.4	0	1	0	0	0	3	1
6.8	0	0	1	0	0	4	1
5.9	0	0	0	1	0	1	2
1.9	1	0	0	1	0	2	2
4.0	0	1	0	1	0	3	2
6.5	0	0	1	1	0	4	2
6.1	0	0	0	0	1	1	3
5.0	1	0	0	0	1	2	3
4.6	0	1	0	0	1	3	3
6.9	0	0	1	0	1	4	3

MINITAB output

```
The regression equation is
Y = 5.21 - 2.07 X2 - 1.13 X3 + 1.27 X4 - 0.150 X6 + 0.925 X7

Predictor        Coef        Stdev      t-ratio          p
Constant       5.2083       0.5851         8.90      0.000
X2            -2.0667       0.6756        -3.06      0.022 ⎫
X3            -1.1333       0.6756        -1.68      0.144 ⎬ treatments
X4             1.2667       0.6756         1.87      0.110 ⎭

X6            -0.1500       0.5851        -0.26      0.806 ⎫
X7             0.9250       0.5851         1.58      0.165 ⎬ blocks

s = 0.8275       R-sq = 83.9%        R-sq(adj) = 70.5%

Analysis of Variance

SOURCE          DF           SS          MS         F          p
Regression       5      21.3883      4.2777      6.25      0.023
Error            6       4.1083      0.6847
Total           11      25.4967

CONTINUE?
SOURCE          DF        SEQ SS
X2               1       10.0278
X3               1        6.2422
X4               1        2.4067
X6               1        1.0004
X7               1        1.7112
```

The estimated treatment effects

The estimated mean differences in treatment responses can be obtained from the estimated coefficients ($\hat{\tau}_2$, $\hat{\tau}_3$, $\hat{\tau}_4$ and $\hat{\beta}_2$ and $\hat{\beta}_3$). Remember that τ_1, and β_2 have been constrained to take value 0.

The estimated mean difference in response between treatment 2 and 1

$$= \hat{\tau}_2 - \tau_1 = -2.0667$$

and the estimated mean difference in response between treatments 3 and 2

$$= \hat{\tau}_3 - \hat{\tau}_2$$
$$= -1.1333 - (-2.0667)$$
$$= 0.9334$$

Similarly $\hat{\tau}_4 - \hat{\tau}_2 = 1.2667 - (-2.0667) = 3.3334$ and so on.

The same results can also be obtained by using GLM commands. This is shown using SAS. The data are held in a file on drive A: that is labelled Block2.dat. The structure is as shown in the printout.

SAS commands

	Objective
`data block2;`	File identifier.
`infile 'a:block2.dat';`	Location of data.
`input Y Treat Block;`	Inputs the three columns of data.
`run;`	
`Proc Print;`	
`run;`	
`Prog GLM;`	Invokes the GLM procedure.
`class Block Treat;`	Declares the two variables as categorical variables.
`model Y = Block Treat / solution;`	Defines the two factor model and asks for coefficients to be printed.
`run;`	

SAS output

Table 10.15 gives the data file.

```
                    General Linear Models Procedure

Dependent Variable: Y

                        Sum of         Mean
Source            DF    Squares        Square     F Value   Pr > F

Model              5    21.38833333    4.27766667    6.25   0.0226
Error              6     4.10833333    0.68472222
Corrected Total   11    25.49666667


         R-Square         C.V.        Root MSE        Y Mean
         0.838868      16.60494       0.827479      4.98333333


Source            DF    Type I SS    Mean Square   F Value   Pr > F

BLOCK              2     2.71166667   1.35583333     1.98    0.2186
TREAT              3    18.67666667   6.22555556     9.09    0.0119


Source            DF    Type III SS  Mean Square   F Value   Pr > F

BLOCK              2     2.71166667   1.35583333     1.98    0.2186
TREAT              3    18.67666667   6.22555556     9.09    0.0119
```

Parameter		Estimate	T for H0: Parameter = 0	Pr > |T|	Std Error of Estimate
INTERCEPT		7.400000000 B	12.65	0.0001	0.58511632
BLOCK	1	−0.925000000 B	−1.58	0.1650	0.58511632
	2	−1.075000000 B	−1.84	0.0058	0.58511632
	3	0.000000000 B	.	.	.
TREAT	1	−1.266666667 B	−1.87	0.1099	0.67563413
	2	−3.333333333 B	−4.93	0.0026	0.67563413
	3	−2.400000000 B	−3.55	0.0120	0.67563413
	4	0.000000000 B	.	.	.

Note that the estimates for the coefficients of the model are not the same in GLM and in the regression approach used earlier because different constraints are imposed. In the regression approach τ_1 and β_1 were constrained to zero whereas in GLM, β_3 and τ_4 were constrained to zero (see outputs). However, the estimates of the differences are the same, as shown:

GLM $\tau_4 - \tau_3 = 0 - 2.40 = 2.40$ $\tau_3 - \tau_2 = -2.4 + 3.333 = 0.9333$
Regression $\tau_4 - \tau_3 = 2.40$ $\tau_3 - \tau_2 = 0.9333$

10.13   Two factor experiments with repeated measures

One very common design used in experimental work in the life sciences is the two factor repeated measures design. Typically n subjects are recruited and randomly allocated to receive one of k treatments (factor 1). Their responses are then monitored at different times (factor 2). For example, in *bioequivalence testing* of two formulations of a given drug, volunteers are recruited to randomly receive one of the two products (e.g. capsule and solution). The blood levels of the drug are

Table 10.15   Data in file block2.dat.

OBS	Y	TREAT	BLOCK
1	4.4	1	1
2	3.3	2	1
3	4.4	3	1
4	6.8	4	1
5	5.9	1	2
6	1.9	2	2
7	4.0	3	2
8	6.5	4	2
9	6.1	1	3
10	5.0	2	3
11	4.6	3	3
12	6.9	4	3

then recorded at different time points. In such testing, the objective of the experiment is usually to test whether the concentration–time profiles are the same. For each patient the profiles may take the form shown in Fig. 10.3.

It may be tempting to compare the individual concentrations at, say, time t_1 by using a test such as the t-test. The same approach would then be used at different time points. This would be incorrect since the overall α-level is not controlled and the question asked, whether the profiles are the same, is not answered. Additionally the measurements at different times are correlated (i.e. the concentration at time t_n is related to that at time t_{n-1} etc.). Several approaches are possible for overcoming these difficulties in the analysis of such serial measurements:

(1)   *Use of summary measures.*
      One approach is to use summary measures. The area under the curve, the slope and t_{max}, the time at which peak maximum is observed, are often used. Those summary measures are then used as if they were raw data. When analysing such data the first step is, therefore, calculation of the summary measure. The values obtained are then analysed by the methods already discussed (e.g. the t-test for two formulations and one factor (formulation) ANOVA for three or more formulations). Often in such bioequivalence studies, the same subjects are given each of the formulations over different periods with a wash-out period in between. This is to reduce the error variance to enable smaller difference to be identified with manageable sample sizes. The period allocation is randomised. Such a trial is called a *cross-over trial* as the subjects are crossed over to receive a different formulation in each period. In such a case, the significance of any period and sequence effects must be tested for. If summary measures are used, the design can then be considered to be a two factor design with formulation and period being the two factors.

(2)   *Use of repeated measures analysis.*
      Instead of using the summary measures, the actual serially correlated data are used.

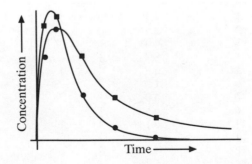

Fig. 10.3   Typical concentration–time profiles observed in bioavailability studies.

The total sum of squares are partitioned into between-subjects sum of squares and within-patients sum of squares. These are in turn subdivided as shown:

Between-Patients SS = Formulation SS + Patients (formulation) SS.
Within-Patients   SS = Time SS + Time × formulation SS + Error SS.
Total   SS = Between-Patient SS + Within-Patients SS.

In practice with bioavailability studies, the wash-out period is chosen based on what is already known about the characteristics of the drug. Therefore carry-over effects are highly unlikely. However, the following example shows how sequence effects are tested for the subsequent analysis of a two-period bioavailability study.

10.13.1   Bioequivalence testing

The data given in Table 10.16 arose from a two-period cross-over study comparing the absorption of an antibiotic in twelve healthy subjects. The area under the plasma concentration time curve (AUC) was used as a summary measure.

Table 10.16 Data from a bioequivalence study of an antibiotic.

Subject	Period	Sequence	Product	AUC (μg h ml^{-1})
1	1	1	1	50.18
1	2	1	2	61.18
2	2	2	1	39.40
2	1	2	2	30.88
3	2	2	1	45.27
3	1	2	2	43.37
4	1	1	1	24.17
4	2	1	2	42.63
5	1	1	1	27.75
5	2	1	2	36.53
6	2	2	1	30.53
6	1	2	2	41.74
7	2	2	1	34.02
7	1	2	2	27.09
8	1	1	1	40.13
8	2	1	2	42.60
9	2	2	1	30.17
9	1	2	2	25.77
10	1	1	1	30.22
10	2	1	2	37.20
11	1	1	1	39.27
11	2	1	2	36.27
12	2	2	1	36.08
12	1	2	2	29.16

The sequence relates to the order in which the subject concerned received the two products. Sequence 1 refers to the products being given in the order 1 and 2 and vice versa for sequence 2.

10.13.2 Testing for carry-over effects

Analysis of cross-over trials is complicated and controversial. Some authors recommend testing for carry-over (sequence) effects before further analyses. This is done by calculating the sum of squares for the sequences and the within-group sum of squares. Using MINITAB GLM command, this is easily done by using the command

```
MTB > GLM AUC = Sequence Subjects Treatment.
```

The program will return the warning that the design is not of full rank. However, the correct sum of squares for the factors sequence and subjects will be returned. The sequence effect can be tested using the F-ratio given by

$$F = \frac{SS(\text{sequence})/1}{SS(\text{subjects})/10} = \frac{124.443}{1105.948/10} = 1.125.$$

This is an F-value from the F-distribution with 1 and 10 degrees of freedom. This value is well outside the critical region and the null hypothesis for absence of sequence effect cannot be rejected. Note that the reduced degrees of freedom (ten) is used to calculate the mean square error.

10.13.3 Testing for treatment effect

The analysis can now proceed with the following commands

```
MTB > GLM AUC = Subject Period Product
```

giving the output shown:

MINITAB output

```
Factor        Levels   Values
Subject          12           1  2  3  4  5  6  7  8  9  10  11  12

Period            2           1  2
Product           2           1  2

Analysis of Variance for AUCInf

Source       DF     Seq SS      Adj SS      Adj MS        F         P
Subject      11     1230.39     1230.39     111.85      4.17     0.016
```

```
Period       1      160.94      160.94      160.94      6.00      0.034
Product      1       30.89       30.89       30.89      1.15      0.308
Error       10      268.07      268.07       26.81
Total       23     1690.30
```

Unusual observations for AUCInf

```
Obs.      AUCInf         Fit    Stdev. Fit      Residual    St. Resid
11       30.5300     37.5900        3.9544       -7.0600        -2.11R
12       41.7400     34.6800        3.9544        7.0600         2.11R
```

R denotes an obs. with a large st. resid.

   The results (see output) show that the null hypothesis of no difference in mean AUC for the two products cannot be rejected ($P = 0.308$) although there was a significant period effect ($P = 0.034$).

10.14   Confidence interval

To estimate the confidence interval for any observed difference in mean AUC for the two products, the following calculations are carried out.

$$\text{Mean difference in AUC for the two products} = (37.87 - 35.60) = 2.27$$

$$95\% \text{ confidence interval} = 2.27 \pm \left[t_{1-\alpha/2}\right]\sqrt{\text{MSE}\left(\frac{1}{n_1} + \frac{1}{n_2}\right)} \qquad (10.21)$$

where MSE is the mean square error from the output and n_1 and n_2 are the sample sizes (12 in each case).

$$95\% \text{ CI} = 2.27 \pm 2.23 \times \sqrt{26.81\left(\frac{1}{12} + \frac{1}{12}\right)}$$

$$= \left[-2.44, \ 6.98\right].$$

   Relative to product A, product B is [($-2.44/37.87$) × 100] or 6.44% less to [(6.98/37.87) × 100] or 18.43% more bioavailable. The interval straddles the 0 point, a result which is consistent with non-rejection of the null hypothesis that the two products are bioequivalent with respect to absorption.
   If a positive sequence effect is observed then the data in the second sequence is ignored and the analysis is restricted to the first half of the data set. In practice this often means repeating the study.

Chapter 11
Diagnostic Tests and Epidemiology

11.1 Objective

In this chapter statistical terminology, concepts and methods associated with diagnostic tests and epidemiological studies are discussed (see Fig. 11.1).

11.2 Diagnostic tests

Diagnostic tests are widely used by health scientists and practitioners for a variety of purposes such as the identification of (1) toxins in foods, (2) abnormalities induced by diseases such as diabetes and infection and (3) changes in physiological states, e.g. pregnancy. The diverse reasons for identifying those changes include: (a) early treatment of diseases to minimise mortality and morbidity (e.g. cancer and upper urinary tract infections), (b) prevention of diseases (e.g. cholesterol testing), and (c) ensuring optimum outcome of a physiological process, (e.g. pregnancy). Whatever the ultimate goal of a diagnostic test, there is a need to define its performance.

In this chapter statistical performance indicators for diagnostic tests are described. Although most diagnostic tests depend on the quantitative measurement of a continuous variable such as urinary sugar level, human chorionic gonadotrophin level, cholesterol level, aflatoxin level and blood pressure, in practice an arbitrary cut-off point is chosen so that the test result is dichotomous, i.e. positive or negative. In this chapter, discussion will be confined to those reduced tests except when method comparison is considered.

11.2.1 Test results

All diagnostic tests occasionally give spurious results. Sometimes they fail to give a positive result when a disease is present (false-negative) or alternatively give a positive result in the absence of the disease (false-positive). Both types of spurious outcomes are undesirable but in some instances it is desirable to err on the side of false-negatives (e.g. where the outcome may determine whether a person faces criminal charges) while in others, false-positives are more acceptable (e.g. when a positive test result will ensure more extensive follow-up of a potentially life-threatening disease).

Consider Table 11.1 which gives hypothetical results for trials of a diagnostic test. Test statistics which can be calculated from the sample results are:

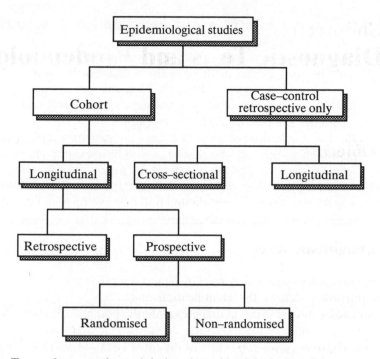

Fig. 11.1 Types of commonly used designs for epidemiological studies.

Table 11.1 Hypothetical results for trials of a diagnostic test. a, b, c and d are integers.

		Disease		Total
		(+)	(−)	
Test result	(+)	a	b	$a + b$
	(−)	c	d	$c + d$
Total		$a + c$	$b + d$	

(1) *Sensitivity* which defines the proportion or percentage of those who should have responded positively to the test actually doing so. The term is also qualitatively defined as *absence of false-negative results.*

(2) *Specificity* which defines the proportion or percentage of those who should have responded negatively to the test actually doing so. The term is also qualitatively defined as *absence of false-positive results.*

(3) *False-negative rate.* There are unfortunately two different definitions for this term:

   (a) the proportion of those with the disease or characteristic who respond negatively to the test, $c/(a + c)$ in Table 11.1, and

   (b)   the proportion of those who respond negatively to the test but have the disease, $c/(c + d)$ in Table 11.1.

(4) *False-positive rate.* Again there are two definitions for this term:

   (a)   the proportion of those without the disease who respond positively to the test, $b/(b + d)$ in Table 11.1, and

   (b)   the proportion of those who respond positively to the test but do not have the disease, $b/(b + a)$ in Table 11.1.

(5) *Positive predictive value* which defines the proportion of all those responding positively to the test who should indeed have responded in this manner (i.e. proportion of true positives among the positive responses).

(6) *Negative predictive value* which defines the proportion of all those responding negatively to the test who should indeed have responded in this manner (i.e. proportion of true negatives among the negative responses).

The test statistics may be given by the following equations:

$$\text{Sensitivity} = a/(a+c) \tag{11.1}$$

$$\text{Specificity} = d/(b+d) \tag{11.2}$$

$$\text{False negative rate} = c/(a+c) \text{ i.e. } 1-(\text{sensitivity}) = \text{definition 1}$$
$$\text{or} = c/(c+d) = \text{definition 2} \tag{11.3}$$

$$\text{False positive rate} = b/(b+d) \text{ i.e. } 1-(\text{specificity}) = \text{definition 1}$$
$$\text{or} = b/(a+b) = \text{definition 2} \tag{11.4}$$

$$\text{Positive predictive value} = a/(a+b) \tag{11.5}$$

$$\text{Negative predictive value} = d/(c+d) \tag{11.6}$$

Example 11.1

Suppose that in 500 consecutive trials of a diagnostic test the results shown in Table 11.2 were obtained. Calculate the test's (1) sensitivity, (2) specificity, (3) false positive rate, (4) false negative rate, (5) positive predictive value and (6) negative predictive value as percentages.

Table 11.2   Test results for a diagnostic test.

		Disease (+)	Disease (−)	Total
Test result	(+)	242	8	250
	(−)	40	210	250
Total		282	218	

Solution

(1)	Sensitivity	$= (242/282) \times 100 = 85.8\%$
(2)	Specificity	$= (210/218) \times 100 = 96.3\%$
(3)	False negative	$= (40/282) \times 100 = 14.2\%$
		or $(40/250) \times 100 = 16\%$
(4)	False positive	$= (8/218) \times 100 = 3.7\%$
		or $(8/250) \times 100 = 3.2\%$
(5)	Positive predictive value	$= (242/250) \times 100 = 96.8\%$
(6)	Negative predictive value	$= (210/250) \times 100 = 84\%$

Note:

- The false negative value

  $$= 1 - (\text{sensitivity})$$
  $$\text{or} = 1 - (\text{negative predictive value})$$

  depending on which definition of false negative value is used. Therefore when reading reports on diagnostic tests or when reporting data on such tests, make sure that the terms are defined and explained.
- Similarly the false positive value

  $$= 1 - (\text{specificity})$$
  $$\text{or} = 1 - (\text{positive predictive value}).$$

- Sensitivity and specificity are unaffected by prevalence while the negative and positive predictive values are.

Q11.1

In a review (*The Medical Letter* (1991) **33**, 40) of rapid diagnostic tests for group A streptococcal pharyngitis it is stated that manufacturers usually claim a *sensitivity* of 90% to 95% and a *specificity* of 95% to 99% for their tests. In *clinical use* the tests' specificity has been higher than 90% while the reported sensitivity has varied between 60% and 95%. What do they mean?

A11.1

They mean that manufacturers of the tests claim that out of every 100 true positive cases tested, 90 to 95 of them will show a positive result on the tests (sensitivity). Of 100 true negative cases tested 95 to 99 will yield a negative result (specificity). In clinical use more than 90% of the tests give negative results for such true-negatives while the positive response rates to true-positive cases have ranged from 60% to 95%.

Q11.2

In a study by Kingdom *et al.* (1991) the performance of a urine test for chorionic gonadotrophin in women with emergency gynaecological problems was investigated with the results given in Table 11.3. Calculate the sensitivity, specificity, positive predictive value and negative predictive value.

Table 11.3 Results of pregnancy tests.

Result of test	Serum chorionic gonadotrophin level above 51 U/L confirmed		Total
	Yes	No	
Positive	78	1	79
Negative	0	51	51
Total	78	52	130

A11.2

Sensitivity = 78/(78 + 0) × 100 = 100%
Specificity = 51/(51 + 1) × 100 = 98%
Positive predictive value = 78/(78 + 1) × 100 = 98.7%.
Negative predictive value = 51/(51 + 0) × 100 = 100%.

Q11.3

How does prevalence of a disease affect a test's (1) sensitivity, (2) specificity, (3) positive predictive value and negative predictive value?

A11.3

Consider an increase in prevalence as shown below:

	Present	Absent
Test (+)	a	b
(−)	c	d

$\xrightarrow{\text{Prevalence increased}}$

	Present	Absent
	$2a$	b
	$2c$	d

Sensitivity $= \dfrac{a}{a+c}$ $\qquad \dfrac{2a}{2a+2c} = \dfrac{a}{a+c}$

Specificity $= \dfrac{b}{b+d}$ $\qquad = \dfrac{b}{b+d}$

Positive predictive value $= \dfrac{a}{a+b}$ $\qquad = \dfrac{2a}{2a+b}$

Negative predictive value $= \dfrac{d}{c+d}$ $\qquad = \dfrac{d}{2c+d}$

Sensitivity and specificity are therefore unaltered by changes in prevalence of the disease. In practice, accurate estimation of the sensitivity of a test will be difficult if the disease is rare. The predictive values are, however, clearly influenced by the prevalence of the disease.

11.2.2   *Bayes' theorem*

In practice, users of a diagnostic test would have data on its sensitivity and specificity and prevalence data on the disease or characteristic being tested for. The required answer is the probability of the disease or characteristic being present given a positive test. Bayes' theorem enables the appropriate calculation to be made.

Bayes' theorem states that given two events A and B

$$P\left(B|A\right) = \frac{P\left(A|B\right)P\left(B\right)}{P\left(A\right)}$$
(11.7)

where $P(B|A)$ is the shorthand for probability of event B given event A has occurred.

Q11.4
What does $P(A|B)$ stand for?

A11.4
Probability of event A given that event B has occurred.
  When applied to a diagnostic test Bayes' theorem can be rewritten as

$$P\left(D+|T+\right) = \frac{P\left(T+|D+\right)P(D+)}{P(T+)}$$
(11.8)

where $P(D+|T+)$ is the positive predictive value, $P(T+|D+)$ is the sensitivity, $P(D+)$ is the prevalence and $P(T+)$ is the probability of a positive test.
  In statistical terminology $P(D+|T+)$, or the positive predictive value, is called a *posteriori* probability; $P(D+)$ or prevalence, a *priori* probability and the ratio $P(T+|D+)/P(T+)$ or the ratio of sensitivity to probability of a positive test, the *likelihood*.

Example 11.2
The manufacturer of a diagnostic test for a particular disease gives its sensitivity as 90% and its specificity as 80. The disease has a prevalence of 1%. What is the probability that a person has the disease given that he has a positive test.

Solution
Using Bayes' theorem

$$P\left(D+|T+\right) = \frac{P\left(T+|D+\right)P(D+)}{P(T+)}$$
(11.8)

Sensitivity = $P(T+|D+)$ = 0.9
Prevalence = $P(D+)$ = 0.01

Considering 100 patients, 1 has the disease and 99 will not. The one person with the disease will be detected with probability 0.9 while 20% of those without the disease will also give a positive test.

$$P(T+) = \frac{0.9 + 99 \times 0.2}{100} = 0.207$$

$$\therefore \quad P(D+|T+) = \frac{0.9 \times 0.01}{0.207} = 0.043 \text{ or } 4.3\%$$

Note: without careful application of Bayes' theorem, many people would give 0.9 as the answer.

An alternative formula which is also used is:

$$\frac{P(D+)}{P(D-1)} \times \frac{P(T+|D+)}{P(T+|D-)} = \frac{P(D+|T+)}{P(D-|T+)} \tag{11.9}$$

where $P(D-1)$ is the prior odds, $P(T+|D-)$ is the likelihood and $P(D-|T+)$ is the posterior odds.

Applying this formula to Example 11.2

$$\frac{0.01}{0.99} \times \frac{0.9}{0.2} = \frac{P(D+|T+)}{P(D-|T+)} = 0.0455$$

$$\therefore \quad P(D+|T+) = \frac{0.0455}{0.0455 + 1} = 0.043 \text{ or } 4.3\%$$

Generalisation of Bayes' theorem

Bayes' theorem can be generalised to the following:

$$P(D+|S) = \frac{P(S|D_1)P(D_1)}{\sum_{j=1}^{n} P(S|D_j)P(D_j)} \tag{11.10}$$

To understand this formula consider the case where $n = 3$

$$P(D_1|S) = \frac{P(S|D_1)P(D_1)}{P(S|D_1)P(D_1) + P(S|D_2)P(D_2) + P(S|D_3)P(D_3)} \tag{11.11}$$

and suppose that D_1, D_2 and D_3 represent three different diseases and S represents a symptom. It can readily be seen that this formula can be used to calculate $P(D_1|S)$, the probability of a person suffering from disease D_1, given that he has the

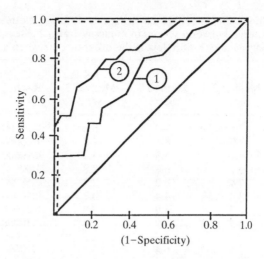

Fig. 11.2 ROC curves. The dotted line represents a perfect test with no false positive or negative results. Curve 2 shows an ROC for a test which is better than a second test whose ROC is shown by curve 1. The diagonal line represents a test with the same rates of false positives and true positives.

symptom, if the prevalence of the three other diseases and the probability of the symptom in the three diseases are known.

Note that the events D_1, D_2 and D_3 are mutually exclusive and exhaustive events in the event space considered and S is any other event.

Bayes' formula in this form is used in the formulation of expert systems for diagnosis of diseases.

11.2.3 *Receiver or relative operating characteristic curves (ROC)*

One increasingly popular method for displaying the ability of a test to discriminate between absence and presence of a particular condition (e.g. disease) is the use of an ROC. This is a plot of the sensitivity of the test against (1 – specificity). Different tests can have their ROC curves plotted on the same graph (see Fig. 11.2).

11.3   Comparing two methods of measurements

New methods of measurements are constantly being introduced to increase ease of use, minimise cost or improve on the performance of existing methods. Before acceptance of a new method, there is a need to compare its performance with the more established methods. For a quantitative response the comparison is usually carried out by taking a series of measurements of the response of interest using the new method and an established method. The paired results are then compared.

Table 11.4 Blood cholesterol levels using two different methods of measurements. Diff1 gives the difference between values in columns 1 and 2. MeanEN gives the mean of the values in columns 1 and 2. DiffNew is the difference between columns 2 and 4.

C1 Method 1 Set 1	C2 Method 2 Set 1	C3 Method 1 Set 2	C4 Method 2 Set 2	C5 Diff1	C6 MeanEN	C7 DiffNew
7.8	7.1	7.7	6.9	0.70000	7.45	0.200000
8.0	7.0	8.1	7.2	1.00000	7.50	−0.200000
5.2	5.1	5.3	5.2	0.10000	5.15	−0.100000
6.7	5.7	6.8	5.8	1.00000	6.20	−0.100000
7.9	7.4	8.0	7.2	0.50000	7.65	0.200000
4.3	3.9	4.4	3.7	0.40000	4.10	0.200000
3.9	3.7	3.9	3.9	0.20000	3.80	−0.200000
3.8	3.5	3.9	3.4	0.30000	3.65	0.100000
3.8	3.8	3.9	4.0	0.00000	3.80	−0.200000
6.6	5.4	6.4	5.5	1.20000	6.00	−0.100000
4.5	3.5	4.4	3.6	1.00000	4.00	−0.100000
6.0	5.5	5.9	5.3	0.50000	5.75	0.200000
5.6	5.2	5.6	5.1	0.40000	5.40	0.100000
4.2	3.4	4.3	3.6	0.80000	3.80	−0.200000
6.2	5.4	6.3	5.2	0.80000	5.80	0.200000
5.7	5.3	5.8	5.4	0.40000	5.50	−0.100000
4.6	4.6	4.4	4.8	0.00000	4.60	−0.200000
4.6	4.8	4.6	4.6	−0.20000	4.70	0.200000
6.3	5.8	6.2	6.1	0.50000	6.05	−0.300000
4.2	5.3	4.6	5.7	1.10000	4.75	−0.400000

To illustrate the recommended approach to evaluating such data, results of a study comparing two methods of blood cholesterol levels will be used. Blood samples were collected from 20 subjects and each sample was measured twice for cholesterol by two different methods, an existing method (Method 1) and a new method, called Method 2. Table 11.4 lists the results.

Step 1
Plot the values obtained with the new method against the current method using the same axes and draw the line of equality. This is shown in Fig. 11.3 using column 1 and 2 data.

Step 2
Calculate the differences between corresponding values obtained using the two methods. The results (C1 − C2) are shown in column 5, labelled Diff1.

Step 3
Plot the observed difference (C5) against the mean of the results [(C1 + C2)/2] obtained using the two methods and show the '*limits of agreement*' or '*the 95% normal range*'. This is shown in Fig. 11.4.

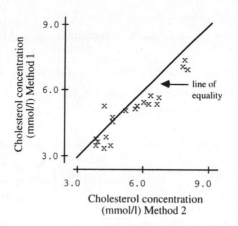

Fig. 11.3   Plot of values obtained using two methods of measurement.

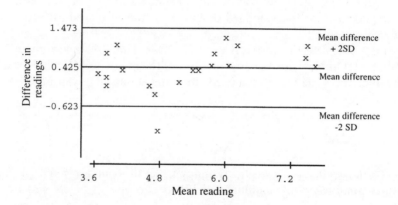

Fig. 11.4   Limits of agreement for the cholesterol data.

If normality assumptions are met, the 95% normal range and the limits of agreement are both approximately given by

$$\text{mean difference} \pm 2 \times \left[\text{standard deviation} \right]$$
$$\left(\text{mean of C5} \right) \quad \pm 2 \times \left[\text{standard deviation of C5} \right]$$

With large sample sizes the value $z_{1-\alpha/2}$ which is 1.96 at 0.05 significance level can be used. With small samples the corresponding $t_{1-\alpha/2}$ from the t-distribution with $(n-1)$ degrees of freedom is used.

In the present example the limits of agreement are given by

$$0.425 \pm 2 \times 0.524 \qquad \text{or} \left[-0.62, \ 1.47 \right].$$

Step 4
Calculate the 95% confidence interval for the mean difference. This is given by

$$\text{Mean difference} \pm 1.96 \times \left[\text{standard error}\right]$$

or   Mean difference $\pm 1.96 \times s/\sqrt{n}$

or   Mean difference $\pm t_{1-\alpha/2}\, s/\sqrt{n}$ where n is the sample size.

In the present example, the 95% confidence interval is given by

$$0.425 \pm 2.093 \times 0.524/\sqrt{20} \qquad \text{or} \left[0.18,\ 0.67\right]$$

The $t_{0.975}$ value from the t-distribution with 19 degrees of freedom is used here because of the small sample size.

Step 5
Calculate and quote the coefficients of repeatability (CR) for both methods. This is equal to twice the standard deviation of the observed differences in replicate measurements.

First calculate the differences (C2 – C4). The values are given in column C7 labelled 'DiffNew' for the new method. If the mean of differences is assumed to be 0 (since the same method is used) then the standard deviation

$$\sqrt{\sum\left(x_i - 0\right)^2 \big/ \left(n-1\right)} = \sqrt{\left(\frac{\sum x_i^2}{n-1}\right)}$$

where x_i are the individual differences listed in column C7. Twice this value gives the *coefficient of repeatability*.

$$\text{CR} = \text{coefficient of repeatability} = 2\sqrt{\left(\frac{\sum x_i^2}{n-1}\right)}$$

For the present example, the data using the new method

$$\text{CR} = 2 \times \sqrt{\left(\frac{0.76}{19}\right)}$$
$$= 0.40$$

MINITAB

The calculations are easily performed using MINITAB. The following commands can be used.

Objective

```
MTB>GPlot C2 C1
```
This produces Fig. 11.3.

```
MTB>Let C5 = C1 - C2
```
This calculates the difference between the corresponding values in columns 1 and 2.

```
MTB>Let C6 = (C1 + C2)/2
```
This calculates the mean of corresponding values in columns 1 and 2.

```
MTB>Let C7 = (C2 - C4)
```
This calculates the difference in replicate values obtained using Method 2.

```
MTB>GPlot C5 C6;
SUBC>yincrement = 3;
SUBC>xincrement = 3;
SUBC>ystart = 3 End = 9;
SUBC>xstart = 3 End = 9.
```
This sequence of commands produces Fig. 11.4.

```
MTB>Describe C5.
```
This produces the output shown.

MINITAB output

	N	MEAN	MEDIAN	TRMEAN	STDEV	SEMEAN
Diff1	20	0.425	0.450	0.467	0.524	0.117

The output enables calculation of the 95% confidence interval and the limits of agreement (see steps 4 and 5).

11.4   Epidemiological studies

Two types of observational studies are widely used in epidemiology including pharmacoepidemiological studies: case-control and cohort studies. Clinical trials are rarely used because in most studies investigating potential adverse effects, those effects are relatively rare. Therefore inordinately large and prohibitively expensive studies are required in order to identify an increased incidence of those adverse effects relative to the background incidence.

The *case-control study* starts with study subjects (cases) who already have the disease of interest and control subjects without the disease. The previous exposures of subjects in both groups are then followed to determine whether the cases show an excess exposure.

The *cohort study*, on the other hand, is one in which a group of subjects exposed to a factor of interest and an unexposed control group are followed over time to determine if they show differences in disease incidence attributable to their different exposures. Cohort studies are by definition usually prospective. However, in a cohort study occupational records may be used to identify past exposures and the

Table 11.5 Strengths and weaknesses of case-control and cohort studies.

Study type	Strengths	Weaknesses
Case-control	Several outcomes can be monitored. Rare diseases can be studied. Relatively inexpensive.	Selection of controls is difficult.
Cohort	Several outcomes can be monitored. Incidence data is readily computed as an outcome. Rarely used drugs can be considered.	Long-term follow-up may be required. Confounding factors may creep in during study to introduce bias.

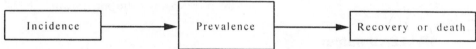

Fig. 11.5 Illustrating the relationship between incidence and prevalence rates.

subjects are then traced forward in time since the exposure to observe subsequent diseases. Such a cohort study is therefore retrospective.

A comparison between case-control and cohort studies can be seen in Table 11.5.

Some terminology

Morbidity is the frequency of illness or disability while *mortality* is the frequency of death.

The *prevalence rate* defines the proportion of a defined group having a particular condition at one point in time. The *incidence rate* on the other hand is the proportion of a defined group developing the condition within a stated period. The relationship between prevalence and incidence rates is shown in Fig. 11.5.

Odds refers to the ratio of the probability of occurrence of an event to that of non-occurrence. For example, if the probability of a patient developing a cough while receiving an angiotensin converting enzyme inhibitor is 0.20, then the odds of this event is $0.20/(1 - 0.20) = 0.25$ (see Table 11.6).

The *odds ratio* is the ratio of two odds. For example, if the odds of developing a disease while receiving a drug and when not receiving it are 0.4 and 0.2 respectively, then the odds ratio is 0.4/0.2 or 2 (see Table 11.6).

In the contingency table given in Table 11.6, the odds ratio is given by $(a/c)/(b/d)$ or ad/bc.

Table 11.6 Contingency table showing disease occurrence with and without exposure to a drug.

		Drug exposure Yes	No	Total
Disease present	Yes	a	c	n_1
	No	b	d	n_2
Total		n_3	n_4	n

11.4.1 Case-control studies

Confidence interval for an odds ratio (Woolf's method)

The odds ratio (OR) is always positive and rarely exceeds 10. Its probability distribution is therefore non-normal with usually encountered sample sizes. The logarithmic transformation $\log_e(\text{OR})$ is often used to produce an approximately normal distribution. Its variance is given by

$$\text{Variance of } \log_e(\text{OR}) = \frac{1}{n}\left(\frac{1}{P_1} + \frac{1}{1-P_1} + \frac{1}{P_2} + \frac{1}{1-P_2}\right) \tag{11.12}$$

where P_1 and P_2 are the probabilities of exposure given the presence or absence of the disease respectively. It is approximated by

$$\text{Variance of } \log_e(\text{OR}) = V\left[\log_e(\text{OR})\right] = \left(\frac{1}{a} + \frac{1}{b} + \frac{1}{c} + \frac{1}{d}\right) \tag{11.13}$$

The confidence interval for $\log_e(\text{OR})$ is therefore given by

$$\log_e(\text{OR}) \pm z_{1-\alpha/2}\left[\sqrt{\left(\frac{1}{a} + \frac{1}{b} + \frac{1}{c} + \frac{1}{d}\right)}\right] \tag{11.14}$$

The 95% confidence interval equals

$$\log_e(\text{OR}) \pm 1.96\left[\sqrt{\left(\frac{1}{a} + \frac{1}{b} + \frac{1}{c} + \frac{1}{d}\right)}\right] \tag{11.15}$$

The confidence interval in the original odds ratio scale is therefore given by $[\text{OR}_L, \text{OR}_U]$ or $[e^{\log_e(\text{OR})_L}, e^{\log_e(\text{OR})_U}]$ where $\log_e(\text{OR})_L$ and $\log_e(\text{OR})_U$ are the lower and upper limits of the $\log_e(\text{OR})$.

Note that the interval $[\text{OR}_L, \text{OR}_U]$ is non-symmetrical about the mean odds ratio. This is shown in Example 11.2.

Example 11.2

Suppose that $a = 80$, $b = 545$, $c = 90$ and $d = 950$, and it is required to calculate the 95% confidence interval for the odds ratio (OR).

Solution

$$\text{OR} = \frac{a/b}{c/d} = \frac{80/545}{90/950} = 1.55$$

$$\log_e(\text{OR}) = 0.4383$$

95% confidence interval for $\log_e(\text{OR})$

$$= \log_e(\text{OR}) \pm z_{1-\alpha/2}\sqrt{\left(\frac{1}{a} + \frac{1}{b} + \frac{1}{c} + \frac{1}{d}\right)}$$

$$= \left\{0.4383 \pm 1.96\left[\sqrt{\left(\frac{1}{80} + \frac{1}{545} + \frac{1}{90} + \frac{1}{950}\right)}\right]\right\}$$

$$= [0.119,\ 0.757] \tag{11.14}$$

95% confidence interval for OR

$$= \left[e^{\log_e(0.119)},\ e^{\log_e(0.757)}\right]$$

$$= [1.13,\ 2.13]$$

Note that the confidence interval is non-symmetrical (see Fig. 11.6).

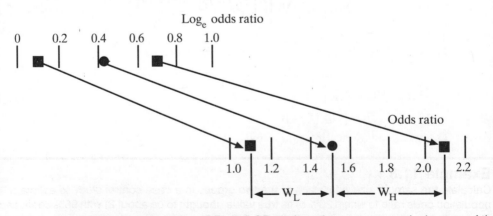

Fig. 11.6 Confidence interval for $\log_e(\text{OR})$ and OR to show the non-symmetrical nature of the interval when the OR is used. ($W_H > W_L$ where W_H represents the interval between the mean value and the upper 95% confidence limit and W_L represents the interval between the mean and the lower 95% confidence limit.) Although the interval for $\log_e(\text{OR})$ is symmetrical. ● = mean value, ■ = lower and upper values.

Calculating sample sizes for estimating an odds ratio in a case-control study

A number of assumptions are made:

(1) Equal sample size n to be used in both groups.
(2) Odds ratio is greater than 1; otherwise interchange groups 'exposed' and 'unexposed'.
(3) One wishes to control the width W_L representing the interval between the mean odds ratio and the lower confidence value.

So, calculating n required to estimate OR to within ε of its true value where

$$\varepsilon = \frac{\left|\hat{OR}_L - OR\right|}{OR} = \frac{W_L}{OR}$$

$$\begin{aligned}\varepsilon OR = OR - \hat{OR}_L &= W_L \\ &= e^{\log_e(OR)} - e^{\log_e(OR)_L} \\ &= e^{\log_e(OR)} - e^{\left\{\log_e(OR) - z_{1-\alpha/2} \times SE\left[\log_e(OR)\right]\right\}} \\ &= OR - ORe^{\left[-z_{1-\alpha/2} SE\left(\log_e(OR)\right)\right]}\end{aligned}$$

$$\begin{aligned}\log_e(1 - \varepsilon) &= -z_{1-\alpha/2} SE\left(\log_e(OR)\right) \\ &= -z_{1-\alpha/2} \times \sqrt{\left\{\frac{1}{n}\left[\frac{1}{P_1(1-P_1)} + \frac{1}{P_2(1-P_2)}\right]\right\}}\end{aligned}$$

Solving

$$n = \frac{z_{1-\alpha/2}^2 \left[\dfrac{1}{P_1(1-P_1)} + \dfrac{1}{P_2(1-P_2)}\right]}{\left[\log_e(1-\varepsilon)\right]^2} \tag{11.16}$$

Example 11.3

Calculate the sample size n for each of the two groups in a case-control study to estimate the population odds ratio to within 20% of its true value (thought to be about 2) with 95% confidence. The control exposure rate is estimated to be 0.6.

Solution

$$\text{Odds ratio (OR)} = \frac{P_1/(1-P_1)}{P_2/(1-P_2)}$$

Rearranging

$$P_1 = \frac{(OR)P_2}{1 - P_2 + (OR)P_2}$$

$$P_2 = 0.6$$

Therefore

$$P_1 = \frac{(2)(0.6)}{1 - 0.6 + (2)(0.6)} = 0.75$$

$$n = \frac{z_{1-\alpha/2}^2 \left[\dfrac{1}{P_1(1-P_1)} + \dfrac{1}{P_2(1-P_2)} \right]}{\left[\log_e(1-\varepsilon) \right]^2}$$

$$= \frac{1.96 \left[\dfrac{1}{0.75(1-0.75)} + \dfrac{1}{0.6(1-0.6)} \right]}{\left[\log_e(1-0.2) \right]^2}$$

$$= 373.95 \approx 374$$

Sample size calculation for hypothesis testing of the odds ratio

The null hypothesis is usually $H_0 : OR = 1$. This is equivalent to $H_0 : P_1 = P_2$ and the alternative hypothesis is $H_1 : P_1 \neq P_2$.

Therefore to calculate the sample size required for hypothesis testing of the odds ratio, the same approach as that used for testing $H_0 = P_1 = P_2$ is appropriate. The appropriate formula is

$$n = \frac{\left\{ z_{1-\alpha/2} \sqrt{\left[2\overline{P}\left(1 - \overline{P}\right) \right]} + z_{1-\beta} \sqrt{\left[P_1\left(1 - P_1\right) + P_2\left(1 - P_2\right) \right]} \right\}^2}{\left(P_1 - P_2 \right)^2} \tag{11.17}$$

where $\overline{P} = (P_1 + P_2)/2$.

In case-control studies, P_2 the control exposure rate is often known with good precision. In this case the following modified expression is used.

$$n = \frac{\left\{ z_{1-\alpha/2} \sqrt{\left[2P_2\left(1 - P_2\right) \right]} + z_{1-\beta} \sqrt{\left[P_1\left(1 - P_1\right) + P_2\left(1 - P_2\right) \right]} \right\}^2}{\left(P_1 - P_2 \right)^2} \tag{11.18}$$

Example 11.4

It is required to evaluate the efficacy of a new vaccine. The available data about vaccination rates in the control subjects is reliable, indicating that 40% are not vaccinated. The disease is severe enough for an odds ratio of 1.5 to be considered an important difference. What sample size should one use in each group to ensure that there is an 80% chance of detecting whether the odds ratio is significantly different from 1 at the 1% level?

Solution

$P_2 = 0.4$; OR $= 1.5$.

Therefore $P_1 = \dfrac{1.5(0.4)}{1 - 0.4 + (1.5)(0.4)} = 0.5$

Since P_2 is known with some certainty Equation 11.19 is used:

$z_{1-\alpha/2} = 2.576$

$z_{1-\beta} = 0.842$

$n = \dfrac{\left[2.576\sqrt{(2 \times 0.4 \times 0.6)} + 0.842\sqrt{(0.5 \times 0.5 + 0.4 \times 0.6)} \right]^2}{(0.5 - 0.4)^2}$

$= 1890.4 \approx 1891$

Note: that if a 5% significance level is acceptable ($z_{1-\alpha/2} = 1.960$), then the sample size required reduces to 380.

11.4.2   Cohort studies

The *risk* of a disease is the probability of its occurrence. The *relative risk* is the ratio of the risk of the disease among those exposed, to the risk among those who are not exposed.

Calculating the confidence interval for a relative risk (Katz method)

Using the same approach as that used with the odds ratio, the confidence interval can be calculated as follows:

The estimated variance of $\log_e(\mathrm{RR})$ is given by

$$\mathrm{Var}\left(\log_e \mathrm{RR}\right) = \frac{b/a}{a+b} + \frac{d/c}{c+d} \tag{11.19}$$

Therefore the $(1 - \alpha/2)\%$ confidence interval for $\log_e$ is given by

$$\log_e\left(\mathrm{RR}\right) \pm z_{1-\alpha/2}\left\{\mathrm{SE}\left[\log_e\left(\mathrm{RR}\right)\right]\right\} \tag{11.20}$$

Having obtained the confidence interval for $\log_e(\mathrm{RR})$ as $[\log_e(\mathrm{RR})_L, \log_e(\mathrm{RR})_U]$ the confidence interval for RR is given by $[e^{\log_e(\mathrm{RR})_L}, e^{\log_e(\mathrm{RR})_U}]$.

Calculating the sample size when estimating a relative risk

Suppose that it is required to estimate the relative risk (RR) to within ε of the true population value. Then the width of the interval W is given by $W_L + W_U$ where W_L = difference between observed relative risk and the lower confidence value RR_L and W_L is the difference between the observed relative risk and the upper confidence value RR_U. As with the odds ratio, the logarithm of the relative risk is used to obtain a probability distribution closer to the normal distribution than the untransformed relative risk.

Using the same approach as used for the odds ratio, the sample size n for each of the exposed and unexposed study group can be shown to be given by

$$n = \frac{z_{1-\alpha/2}^2 \left[\frac{(1-P_1)}{P_1} + \frac{(1-P_2)}{P_2}\right]}{\left[\log_e(1-\varepsilon)\right]^2} \tag{11.21}$$

Attributable risk

The incidence rate (I_r) of a disease in a group exposed to a risk factor is made up of two components: I_e, the incidence rate due to exposure and I_o, the incidence rate due to other factors.

$$I_r = I_e + I_o \tag{11.22}$$

The *attributable risk* (AR) is the excess incidence rate among those exposed to the risk factor (i.e. $I_r - I_o$). The term is also used for the ratio $(I_r - I_o)/I_r$.

$$AR = \frac{I_r - I_o}{I_r} = \frac{I_r/I_o - I_o/I_o}{I_r/I_o} = \frac{RR-1}{RR} \tag{11.23}$$

assuming $RR \geq 1$.

Given a contingency table as shown in Table 11.7.

Table 11.7 Layout of contingency table.

		Disease +	Disease −	Total
Risk factor	+	a	b	$a+b$
	−	c	d	$c+d$
Total		$a+c$	$b+d$	$a+b+c+d$

The estimated relative risk (RR) is given by

$$\hat{RR} = \frac{a/(a+b)}{c/(c+d)} = \frac{a(c+d)}{c(a+b)}$$

(11.24)

$$\hat{AR} = \frac{\hat{RR}-1}{\hat{RR}} = \frac{ad-bc}{ac+ad}$$

(11.25)

For a prospective (cohort study) the variance of AR is given by

$$V(AR) = \frac{cn\left[ad(n-c)+bc^2\right]}{(a+c)^3(c+d)^3}$$

(11.26)

where $n = a + b + c + d$.

Confidence interval for AR

The $(1 - \alpha/2)$ confidence interval is therefore given by

$$AR \pm z_{1-\alpha/2}\left[SE(AR)\right]$$

(11.27)

where SE(AR), the standard error of AR is given by $\sqrt{[V(AR)]}$ and $z_{1-\alpha/2}$ is the z value corresponding to the significance level α required. At $\alpha = 0.05$, $z_{1-\alpha/2}$ is equal to 1.960.

Sometimes the AR, also called the excess risk, is expressed in terms of a given population size (N) using the definition $AR = (I_r - I_o)N$ where $I_e = a/(a + b)$ and $I_o = c/(c + d)$. The attributable risk is then reported as a number per N subjects. For example, if $N = 10\,000$, $a = 12$, $b = 9500$, $c = 5$ and $d = 9800$ then

$$AR = \left[12/(12+9500)-5/(5+9800)\right] \times 10,000$$

or 7.5 per 10 000.

11.4.3 Logit analysis

Logit analysis is used in comparative studies to estimate the effect of a risk factor on a dichotomous outcome or response variable as measured by the odds ratio. The method is particularly useful for simultaneously adjusting for many confounding variables.

Logit analysis is analogous to analysis of covariance in that it achieves with categorical outcome variables what the latter achieves with continuous variables.

Both methods estimate treatment effects after adjusting for one or more confounding variables.

A linear regression model for ANCOVA can be written as with a single confounding variable X and a dichotomous risk variable R (i.e. $R = 1$ when risk is present and 0 when absent) can be written as

$$Y = \alpha + \gamma R + \beta X + \varepsilon \qquad (11.28)$$

If Y is not a continuous variable but is dichotomous (e.g. disease present or absent; adverse reaction present or absent) then the linear regression given has to be modified because Y can only take values ranging from 0 to 1 while the right-hand side is not and the error term ε is dichotomous.

The Y transformation most commonly used is the *logit transform* of ρ, the probability that the response $Y = 1$ given the pair of R and X values.

The logit transformation uses $\log_e$ (odds) as the response variable to yield the *logit model*,

$$\log_e\left[\frac{P}{(1-P)}\right] = \alpha + \gamma R + \beta X + \varepsilon \qquad (11.29)$$

The logit transform can now take values in the range $[-\infty, \infty]$. It can be shown that the estimate of γ using logit analysis can be used to estimate the odds ratio given by $\exp(\gamma)$. The logit model assumes that the odds ratio is constant for all values of X. In other words, in the presence ($R = 1$) and absence ($R = 0$) of the risk factor (R) the response can be represented by two parallel lines

$$\log_e\left[\frac{P}{(1-P)}\right] = (\alpha + \gamma) + \beta X \qquad (11.30)$$

and

$$\log_e\left[\frac{P}{(1-P)}\right] = \alpha + \beta X \qquad (11.31)$$

with γ representing the distance between the two intercepts or two lines.

To estimate the parameters α, γ and β, an iterative procedure called the *maximum likelihood method* is usually resorted to.

Logistic regression

To estimate the parameters (α, γ and β) of the logit model, an iterative procedure, *maximum likelihood*, is commonly used. The analysis assumes that the observations are independent binomial (or Bernoulli) variables.

An alternative estimation procedure which is useful when the experimental units fall into groups when classified by the risk and confounding variables is *logistic regression*, a non-iterative linear regression procedure. While the procedure generally requires a categorical X variable, it can be applied when a numerical X variable is set at different levels and replications are available at each of those levels. For this reason logistic regression is often used in bioassays. The regression model is also modified to

$$\log_e\left[\frac{p}{(1-p)}\right] = \alpha + \gamma R + \beta X + \varepsilon \tag{11.32}$$

where p is the proportion of experimental units showing a 'success' or positive response. The error terms ε in this model have unequal variances and weighted linear regression is used with weights (W) given by

$$W = np(1-p) \tag{11.33}$$

where n is the number of replications in the group with a given pair of R and X values. Most computer packages allow specification of weights as a subcommand to the regression command.

Logit analysis in case-control studies

Logit analysis may also be applied to control studies by interchanging the role of the risk and outcome factors. Remember that in case-control studies the outcome is known already and the objective is to work out the probability of being in the group exposed to the dichotomous risk factor given the observed outcome.

If P' represents the probability of the risk factor being present given the outcome, Y, and the confounding variable, X, the case-control logit model can then be written as

$$\log_e\left[\frac{P'}{(1-P')}\right] = \alpha + \gamma R + \beta X \tag{11.34}$$

γ, the log of the odds ratio and hence the odds ratio ($\exp(\gamma)$), can then be estimated as for cohort studies. The use of the cohort model is acceptable for analysing case-control data if the cases and controls are selected from their respective populations without significant bias (i.e. independently of the risk and confounding factors).

As with linear regression, model adequacy should be checked by performing appropriate goodness-of-fit tests. Interactions between variables R and X is tested for by introducing a new variable RX so that the model then becomes

$$\log_e\left[\frac{P'}{(1-P')}\right] = \alpha + \gamma R + \beta_1 X + \beta_2[RX] \tag{11.35}$$

and testing the null hypothesis $H_0: \beta_2 = 0$.

To deal with multiple confounding factors $(X_1, X_2, \ldots, X_K)$ the model can be simply modified to

$$\log_e \left[\frac{P}{(1-P)} \right] = \alpha + \gamma R + \beta_1 X_1 + \beta_2 X_2 + \ldots + \beta_K X_K \tag{11.36}$$

where P is the probability of the dichotomous outcome taking a value of 1 given a set of $R_1, X_1, X_2 \ldots, X_K$ values. If the confounding variable is categorical with g categories $(g > 2)$ this can be represented by $(g - 1)$ indicator or dummy X variables. Each takes the value 1 if the response datum corresponds to the level indicated by the indicator variable and 0 otherwise.

11.4.4   Log-linear models

Log-linear analysis is used when the risk, outcome and confounding variables are all categorical and can therefore be represented in a contingency table (see Chapter 9). In the log-linear model the logarithm of the expected cell count in the contingency table is expressed as a *linear* function of parameters representing variables and their interactions. For example, in a 2×2 contingency table if i represents the level of the dichotomous outcome variable, j represents the level of treatments $(j = 1$ or $2)$ and m_{ij} represents the corresponding expected cell count then the log-linear model can be written as

$$\log_e m_{ij} = U + U_{i(Y)} + U_{j(R)} + U_{ij(YR)} \tag{11.37}$$

where U is a constant, $U_{i(Y)}$ is a parameter depending on i only, $U_{j(R)}$, a parameter depending on j only and $U_{ij(YR)}$, a parameter measuring the association between Y and R. This model is called the *saturated model* because for a 2×2 contingency table (i.e. of size 4) only four parameters are permissible. In the absence of a treatment or risk factor effect, the log-linear model reduces to the no-treatment effect or independence model

$$\log_e m_{ij} = U + U_{i(Y)} + U_{j(R)} \tag{11.38}$$

The use of log-linear models for analysing a 2×2 contingency table provides no more information than the usual χ^2 test for independence and the crude odds ratio. However, with higher order contingency tables, log-linear analysis provides significant advantage over the simpler analyses because it gives access to models intermediate between the independence and the saturated models. The interested reader is referred to Agresti (1990).

Chapter 12
Survival Analysis

12.1 What is survival analysis?

Survival analysis refers to a group of statistical methods used for analysing data in which the outcome variable is time until occurrence of an event (e.g. time to death, time to recovery, time to relapse, time to product failure).

12.2 What are censored data?

One of the key problems to be addressed in survival analysis is the fact that often, we do not have the exact survival time. Instead, we know that the subject or object has survived at least up to a given time. Typically, we may know how many subjects have survived until the end of, say, a one-year study but we do not know how much longer they may survive. Alternatively, we may lose subjects to follow-up during the course of a study. Such incomplete data are referred to as *censored data*.

Figure 12.1 shows types of censored data which may arise during a survival study.

12.3 What is the survivor function?

The survivor function, usually denoted as $S(t)$, gives the probability that a person survives longer than some specified time t. At the start of the study $S(t) = 1$ and at time infinity, $S(t) = 0$ because $S(t)$ is on a probability scale. The survivor function is a step function since failure can only assume two states, failure or no failure. In theoretical work, survivor functions are approximated by smooth continuous functions such as the exponential function.

12.4 What is a hazard function?

The hazard function, usually denoted by $h(t)$, gives the instantaneous potential failure *rate* at time t given that the subject has survived until time t. For this reason, $h(t)$ is also referred to as the conditional failure rate.

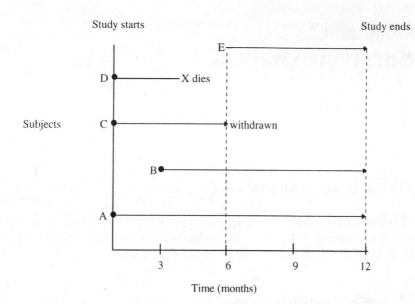

Fig. 12.1   Survival data for five patients to illustrate censoring. Subject A shows a censored survival time. We know that he survived for at least 12 months. Subject B enters the study at 3 months and his survival time is also censored, this time with a survival time of 9 months. Subject C withdraws from the study at 6 months. The censored survival time is now 6 months. Subject D provides a complete survival time of 3 months. Subject E contributes a censored survival time of 6 months.

$$h(t) = \frac{P(t \leq T < t + \Delta t / T \geq t)}{\Delta t} \qquad \text{as } \Delta t \text{ tends to zero}$$

The hazard function may take any positive value.

12.5   What are the objectives in survival analysis?

Survival analysis may be used to:

(1)   Investigate factors which affect survival time (e.g. treatments or diet or stress).
(2)   Compare survivor and/or hazard functions.
(3)   Estimate survivor and/or hazard functions.

The classical approach for analysing survival data with censoring is the Kaplan-Meier method illustrated in Table 12.1.

Table 12.1 Kaplan-Meier survival analysis – calculating survival probabilities.

Subject	Drug	Time (months)	Subject status	n	m	q	$\hat{S}(t)$	
		0		10	0	0	1	
1	1	5	Died	10	2	0	$1 \times 8/10$	$= 0.8000$
2	1	5	Died					
3	1	10	Died	8	1	1	$0.8 \times 7/8$	$= 0.7000$
4	1	16	Died	6	1	0	$0.7 \times 5/6$	$= 0.5833$
5	1	18	Died	5	1	0	$0.5833 \times 4/5 = 0.4667$	
6	1	20	Died	4	1	0	$0.4667 \times 3/4 = 0.3500$	
7	1	10*	Lost					
8	1	24*	Alive	3	0	3	$0.3500 \times 3/3 = 0.3500$	
9	1	24*	Alive					
10	1	24*	Alive					
11	0	3	Died	10	1	0	$1 \times 9/10$	$= 0.9000$
12	0	5	Died	9	1	0	$0.9 \times 8/9$	$= 0.8000$
13	0	6	Died	8	2	0	$0.8 \times 6/8$	$= 0.6000$
14	0	6	Died					
15	0	7	Died	6	1	0	$0.6 \times 5/6$	$= 0.5000$
16	0	8	Died	5	1	0	$0.5 \times 4/5$	$= 0.4000$
17	0	12	Died	4	1	1	$0.4 \times 3/4$	$= 0.3000$
18	0	12*	Lost	3	0	3	$0.3 \times 3/3$	$= 0.3000$
19	0	24*	Alive					
20	1	24*	Alive					

Drug: 1 ≡ drug, 2 ≡ placebo; n = number of patients at risk at beginning of interval; m = number of patients dying at time point shown; q = number censored during interval starting at time point shown; $\hat{S}(t)$ = estimated survival probability; * = censored.

12.6 Modelling survival data

As indicated in Section 12.1, one of the uses of survival analysis is to investigate whether survival is affected by variables such as social deprivation, treatment received or some biochemical marker. Survival proportion is then used as the response variable with the others as the predictor variables.

Recall that in multiple linear regression, the response or y variable is modelled as a function of two or more responses or x variables. An example could be:

$$y = a_0 + a_1 x_1 + a_2 x_2$$

The linear regression coefficient (e.g. a_1) then gives an estimate of how much y would change per unit change of the corresponding x variable (e.g. x_1).

In survival analysis, the response is the proportion surviving while the predictor or x variables could be the same as in multiple linear regression (e.g. treatment, dose level, etc.).

$$S(t) = b_0 + b_1 x_1 + b_2 x_2$$

The regression coefficient (e.g. b_1) in this case, enables the calculation of the hazard ratio (HR) by using the relationship $HR = e_1^b$.

Chapter 13
Confidence Intervals and Sample Sizes

13.1 Confidence intervals

13.1.1 What is a confidence interval?

Suppose that during the quality control of a batch of tablets, a sample of 20 tablets is taken and two are found to be defective. If a further sample of 20 tablets is examined, then it is more than likely that the number of defective tablets found will be different to two even if the batch actually contained 10% defectives. With any particular estimate of the percentage of defective tablets in the batch, it would be useful if one could give some indication of the reliability of that estimate. The confidence interval is used to do this. The 95% confidence interval, for example, is the interval which, when calculated repeatedly will in the long run include the true population mean 95% of the time. Given any single 95% confidence interval, there is therefore a 95% chance that it will include the mean.

Figure 13.1 illustrates this concept further. Twenty-five confidence intervals were simulated from a normal distribution with a mean of 10 and a variance of 0.05^2. It can be seen that even with only 25 simulations, the observed value closely approaches the theoretical 95% value. The confidence interval can, just like the significance level, be altered to say, a 99% confidence interval. The 99% confidence interval is wider than the 95% interval since the requirement is in this instance that 99% of the intervals should include the true population mean.

13.1.2 Confidence intervals and hypothesis testing

In many studies, the objective is to determine the size of any difference in response between groups rather than simply to identify whether or not the difference is statistically significant. Confidence intervals define the range of values within which the difference may fall.

13.1.3 Calculating a confidence interval

Recall that a confidence interval is the range of values which is expected to include the estimate concerned with a level of certainty defined by the confidence level.

Suppose that the parameter of interest is the population mean. A sample is drawn and the sample mean calculated as an estimate of the population mean. To be able to define a confidence interval one will therefore require to know the distributional characteristics of the statistic concerned, the mean in this case.

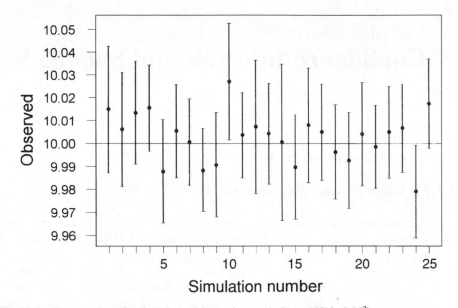

Fig. 13.1 Twenty-five simulated confidence intervals from N(10, 0.05^2).

It is intuitively obvious that if the sample size increases then the estimate of any population parameter will increase in precision. Indeed, if the variance of a given population is σ^2 then the mean, calculated from samples of size n, will have a variance of σ^2/n and a standard deviation of $\sigma/\sqrt{n}$. This standard deviation is called the standard error (SE) of the statistic concerned (the mean in this case). If it is known that the sample mean follows a normal distribution then the confidence interval CI is given by

$$\text{CI} = \bar{x} \pm \left[Z_{1-\alpha/2}\right]\left[\text{SE}\right] \tag{13.1}$$

where $\text{SE} = \sigma/\sqrt{n}$ and where $Z_{1-\alpha/2}$ is the critical value at the appropriate significance level α.

For example, at an α level of 0.05, $Z_{1-\alpha/2} = 1.96$ (Appendix 1). Therefore the 95% confidence interval is given by

$$\text{CI} = \bar{x} \pm 1.96 \times \left[\text{SE}\right] \tag{13.2}$$

If the distribution of the sample mean is the t-distribution then the 95% confidence interval is given by

$$\text{CI} = \bar{x} \pm t_{1-\alpha/2} \times \left[\text{SE}\right] \tag{13.3}$$

If the sample size is say 5, then the $t_{1-\alpha/2}$ with $\alpha = 0.05$ is equal to 2.571 (Appendix 2). Therefore the confidence interval is given by

$$CI = \bar{x} \pm 2.571 \times \left[SE \right] \qquad (13.4)$$

Generally, therefore, in order to calculate a confidence interval for a parameter estimate we would use the following formula

$$CI = \begin{bmatrix} \text{Estimate} \\ \text{e.g. mean} \end{bmatrix} \pm \begin{bmatrix} \text{Critical value from} \\ \text{appropriate distribution} \end{bmatrix} \times \begin{bmatrix} \text{Standard error} \\ \text{of the estimate} \end{bmatrix} \qquad (13.5)$$

Example 13.1
Analysis of ten milk samples gave a mean calcium content of 120 ± 10 mg (mean ± SD). Calculate the 95% confidence interval for the mean calcium content of the milk.

Solution
The calcium content of the milk is assumed to be normally distributed. Since the sample is small, the sampling distribution of the mean is expected to follow a t-distribution with $(n-1)$ or 9 degrees of freedom. The critical value at an $\alpha = 0.05$ significance level is 2.262 (Appendix 2). The standard error (standard deviation of the mean) is $s/\sqrt{n}$ or $10/\sqrt{10}$ in this example. The 95% confidence interval is therefore given by

$$\bar{x} \pm \left[t_{1-\alpha/2} \right] \left[SE \right] \qquad \text{or} \qquad 120 \pm 2.262 \times 10/\sqrt{10} \qquad \text{or} \qquad \left[112.85,\ 127.15 \right]$$

Example 13.2
In a clinical trial of two anti-inflammatory compounds, 32 and 22% of the patients developed some gastro-intestinal disturbance in the two groups of 50 patients each. Calculate the 95% confidence interval for the difference in the two population proportions.

Solution
The difference in sample proportion $= (P_1 - P_2) = 0.32 - 0.22 = 0.10$.

The standard error is given by

$$SE = \sqrt{\left[\frac{P_1(1-P_1)}{n_1} + \frac{P_2(1-P_2)}{n_2} \right]} \qquad (13.6)$$

or

$$\sqrt{\left[\frac{0.32(0.68)}{50} + \frac{0.22(0.78)}{50} \right]} = 0.0864$$

The critical value in the standard normal distribution at $\alpha = 0.05$ is 1.96. Therefore the 95% confidence interval is given by

$$\left[0.10 \pm 1.96 \times 0.0864 \right] \qquad \text{or} \qquad \left[-0.069,\ 0.269 \right]$$

13.1.4 Non-parametric or distribution-free confidence intervals

Parametric tests assume that the data are drawn from specific distributions with the normal distribution being the most common. If an estimate, of say, a population mean, μ, is made by calculating the mean $(\bar{x})$ of a sample drawn from that population, then one can make an assessment of how close the point estimate $(\bar{x})$ is to μ. As discussed in the preceding sections, this assessment is done by calculating a confidence interval. This interval is only valid if the assumption made about the distribution of the data is correct.

With distribution-free methods no rigid assumption is made about the distribution of the data. This, therefore, presents an immediate problem since by definition no parameters are defined for the underlying distributions. It is obvious that a different approach is required for calculating distribution-free confidence intervals. The following text illustrates how such intervals can be calculated. Except for the simplest tests involving small sizes, computers are required to reduce the tediousness of performing those calculations. With MINITAB such calculations form an integral part of the commands used to perform the simpler non-parametric tests as shown in Example 13.3.

Example 13.3
The data set given in Table 13.1 will be used to illustrate the calculation of distribution-free confidence intervals. The data are assumed to have been saved in columns C1 to C4 of a MINITAB worksheet.

Table 13.1 Prothrombin times (in seconds).

Control subjects	9	10	11	12	12	13	14	15	16	16	18	18
Patients pre-treatment	20	21	21	22	22	23	23	23	24	24	24	25
Patients post-treatment	14	16	15	17	11	19	22	17	19	23	24	23
Difference	6	5	6	5	11	4	1	6	5	1	0	2

Solution

Confidence interval for a median
The median prothrombin time for the control subjects is given by $(13 + 14)/2$ or 13.5 seconds. To calculate the 95% confidence interval, the critical values associated with the sign test are used. For a sample size of 12, the critical value at the 5% significance level for a two-sided test is 2 (Appendix 9). To obtain the 95% confidence interval one simply deletes the two more extreme values at either end of the ordered data set (i.e. 9 and 10 at the lower end and 18 and 18 at the upper end). The 95% confidence interval is therefore [11, 16].

To calculate the 95% confidence interval one simply issues the command: MTB> Sinterval C1. The output is shown below. MINITAB uses the binomial theorem to calculate the interval; hence the slight discrepancy with the interval calculated above.

MINITAB output

```
SIGN CONFIDENCE INTERVAL FOR MEDIAN

                                ACHIEVED
       N     MEDIAN          CONFIDENCE     CONFIDENCE INTERVAL      POSITION
C1     12     13.50             0.8540         (12.00, 16.00)              4
                                0.9500         (11.26, 16.00)            NLI
                                0.9614         (11.00, 16.00)              3
```

Confidence interval for a matched-pairs difference

Suppose that a 95% confidence interval for the mean difference in the patients' prothrombin time is required. The hypothesis test appropriate for analysing the data is the Wilcoxon's matched pairs or signed rank test. Therefore one looks up the appropriate critical value for that test (Appendix 8). With a sample size of 12 pairs and a significance level α of 0.05, the critical value is 13.

The possible number of pairwise averages which can be calculated as given by $n(n + 1)$ where n is the number of pairs studied. With $n = 12$ the number of possibilities is therefore 78. These are shown by ordering the differences, in pre- and post-treatment prothrombin times, shown in the last row of the table and arranging them in the form of the square matrix shown in Table 13.2. The 14th smallest mean difference is 2.5 and the 14th largest mean difference is 6. Therefore the 95% confidence interval is given by [2.5, 6].

Table 13.2　Matrix of mean differences.

	0	1	1	2	4	5	5	5	6	6	6	11
11	5.5	6	6	6.5	7.5	8	8	8	8.5	8.5	8.5	11
6	3	3.5	3.5	4	5	5.5	5.5	5.5	6	6	6	
6	3	3.5	3.5	4	5	5.5	5.5	5.5	6	6		
6	3	3.5	3.5	4	5	5.5	5.5	5.5	6			
5	2.5	3	3	3.5	4.5	5	5	5				
5	2.5	3	3	3.5	4.5	5	5					
5	2.5	3	3	3.5	4.5	5						
4	2	2.5	2.5	3	4							
2	1	1.5	1.5	2								
1	1/2	1	1									
1	1/2	1										
0	0											

To compute the 95% confidence interval simply issue the command MTB> WINTERVAL C4. Note that C4 contains the differences obtained by subtracting post-treatment prothrombin times from the pre-treatment values.

MINITAB output

```
                    ESTIMATED           ACHIEVED
           N         MEDIAN            CONFIDENCE      CONFIDENCE INTERVAL
C2-C3     12          4.25               94.5              (2.50, 6.00)
```

Confidence interval for difference between two medians

Table 13.1 gives the prothrombin time for control subjects and a group of pre-treatment patients. An appropriate test for whether the median prothrombin times are different for the two groups is the Mann-Whitney U test. Suppose that one requires the 95% confidence interval for an observed difference. The first step would be to obtain the appropriate critical value. With a sample size of 12 in each group the critical value at $\alpha = 0.05$ is 37.

The next step is to calculate all pairwise comparisons. There are $n_1 \times n_2$ such comparisons or 144 in this example. n_1 and n_2 are the sample sizes for the two groups. This is shown in the matrix given in table 13.3 with the scores arranged in numerical order.

Table 13.3 Pairwise differences in Mann-Whitney U test.

	20	21	21	22	22	23	23	23	24	24	24	25
18	2	3	3	4	4	5	5	5	6	6	6	7
18	2	3	3	4	4	5	5	5	6	6	6	7
16	4	5	5	6	6	7	7	7	8	8	8	9
16	4	5	5	6	6	7	7	7	8	8	8	9
15	5	6	6	7	7	8	8	8	9	9	9	10
14	6	7	7	8	8	9	9	9	10	10	10	11
13	7	8	8	9	9	10	10	10	11	11	11	12
12	8	9	9	10	10	11	11	11	12	12	12	13
12	8	9	9	10	10	11	11	11	12	12	12	13
11	9	10	10	11	11	12	12	12	13	13	13	14
10	10	11	11	12	12	13	13	13	14	14	14	15
9	11	12	12	13	13	14	14	14	15	15	15	16

The 37 lowest values and the 37 highest values are then deleted from the list to give the confidence interval [7, 11].

This interval is calculated by MINITAB after issuing the command MTB> MANN-WHITNEY C2 C1

MINITAB output

```
Mann-Whitney Confidence Interval and Test

PreTreat  N = 12    Median = 23.000
Control   N = 12    Median = 13.500
Point estimate for ETA1-ETA2 is 9.000
95.4 pct c.i. for ETA1-ETA2 is (6.999, 11.000)
W = 222.0
Test of ETA1 = ETA2 vs. ETA1 n.e. ETA2 is significant at 0.0000
The test is significant at 0.0000 (adjusted for ties)
```

Note: Confidence intervals are usually constructed in association with a specific hypothesis test. Therefore the first step is to identify which test is appropriate for the data being analysed.

13.2   The power of a hypothesis test

Consider the following hypothesis test about the mean of a population (μ)

$H_0 : \mu = \mu_0$ i.e. the mean is equal to μ_0.
$H_1 : \mu = \mu_1$ i.e. the mean is equal to μ_1.
or $\mu > \mu_0$ some value greater than μ_0.

Let Fig. 13.2 represent the probability curves for the sample means $\bar{x}_0$ and $\bar{x}_1$.

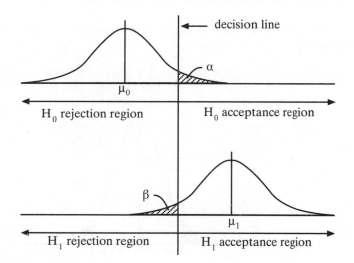

Fig. 13.2   Probability density curves for the sample means $\bar{x}_0$ and $\bar{x}_1$ (upper and lower curves respectively).

If an observed sample mean falls in the α region then H_0 will be rejected. It is obvious that on repeated testing the risk of falsely rejecting H_0 is given by the α-value since the α region is under the probability density curve for $\bar{x}_0$. If the population mean were really μ_1 with a sampling distribution as shown in the lower curve, then β gives the probability of accepting H_0 when it is false since the β region falls in the H_0 acceptance region. The unshaded part of the lower curve equals $(1 - \beta)$ since the curve is a probability density curve. This region therefore gives the probability of rejecting H_0 at the fixed α-value when the population mean is really μ_1 with a sampling distribution shown by the lower curve. For this reason $(1 - \beta)$ is called the *power* of the hypothesis test.

13.3   Sample size calculations

13.3.1   Why calculate sample sizes?

From the discussion on power calculations, it is obvious that a sample size which is too small will carry with it an unacceptable risk of accepting a null hypothesis when it is in fact false. A sample which is larger than required is wasteful of resources and may reveal a statistically significant difference which is of no practical significance. Note in particular that two broad types of calculations are used: those required for estimating population parameters and those required for hypothesis testing.

13.3.2   Sample size calculations for estimation

Figure 13.3 illustrates the items to be considered when estimating the mean of a normally distributed variable.

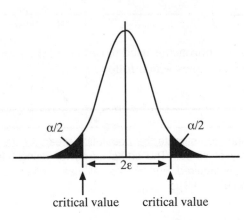

Fig. 13.3 Values which are required when calculating sample sizes for parameter estimation.

The information that is required for calculating samples sizes in connection with parameter estimation are:

(1) The confidence level required for the estimate (i.e. specify α).
(2) The precision required (i.e. specify ε).
(3) Some estimate of the population standard deviation (σ). If this is not available, use one fourth of the expected range to obtain a conservative sample size (i.e. one which errs on the side of being larger than required).
(4) For differences in population parameters, some estimate of their value, perhaps obtained from previous studies.

13.3.3   *Derivation of formulae for calculating sample sizes*

To illustrate how formulae for calculating sample sizes are arrived at, suppose that one wishes to calculate the sample size required for estimating the mean (μ) of a population to within ε, expressed in the same units as μ, with $100(1 - \alpha)\%$ confidence. For a normally distributed variable or with large sample sizes the 95% confidence (95% CI) for the mean is given by

$$95\% \ CI = \bar{x} \pm z_{1-\alpha/2} \frac{s}{\sqrt{n}} \tag{13.7}$$

where $\bar{x}$ is the sample estimate of μ. The critical z-value at a significance level of α is $z_{1-\alpha/2}$. The sample standard deviation is s and n is the sample size. This interval is given by 2ε as shown in Fig. 13.3.

Therefore

$$z_{1-\alpha/2} \frac{2}{\sqrt{n}} = \varepsilon \tag{13.8}$$

$$n = \left(\frac{z_{1-\alpha/2} s}{\varepsilon} \right)^2 \tag{13.9}$$

The same basic approach is used to obtain all the formulae shown in Table 13.4 and used in the examples which follow.

Example 13.3

Suppose that one wishes to estimate the population mean for the vitamin E content (μg per 100g) of a new variety of cereal. The sample size for doing this to within 0.05μg with a confidence level of 99% is required. Perform the calculation given that an initial screen indicates that the standard deviation is 0.3μg.

Solution

The equation to use is

$$n = \left(\frac{z_{1-\alpha/2}}{\varepsilon} \right)^2$$

$$= \left[\frac{(2.576)(0.3)}{0.05} \right]^2 \approx 238 \tag{13.10}$$

where s is the sample standard deviation, $z_{1-\alpha/2}$ is the critical z-value at α significance level and ε is the magnitude of maximum deviation from the mean expressed in the same units. The critical value 2.576 is obtained from Appendix 1.

Example 13.4

In the above example what sample size would one require if one had no estimate of the standard deviation?

Solution

One would need to estimate the range (e.g. $4\,\mu g$) and use one fourth of this for our standard deviation.

$$n = \left[\frac{(2.57)(1)}{(0.05)}\right]^2 = 2642 \text{ (an almost impossible task).}$$

On the other hand if one is willing to accept a precision of $\pm 1\,\mu g$, then

$$n = \left[\frac{(2.57)(1)}{1}\right]^2 = 7$$

a much more manageable number.

13.3.4 Sample size for estimating a population proportion (π)

(a)   To within x percentage points of the true value π (see Fig. 13.4)

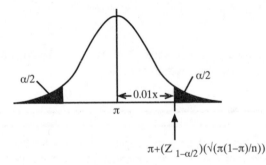

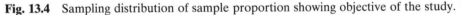

Fig. 13.4   Sampling distribution of sample proportion showing objective of the study.

The sample size (n) can be calculated using the equation

$$n = \frac{z_{1-\alpha/2}^2 P(1-P)}{(0.01x)^2} \tag{13.11}$$

In the absence of a better estimate use $\pi = 0.5$ since this gives a conservative n value, i.e. the n value will tend to be on the safe side (overestimated). $z_{1-\alpha/2}$ is the critical z-value corresponding to a two-sided significance probability α.

Example 13.5

Suppose that we wish to estimate the proportion of children with dental caries from a random sample of children to within 5 percentage points of the true value π with 99% confidence.

Solution

$$n = \frac{(2.58)^2(0.5)(1-0.5)}{(0.01 \times 5)^2} = \approx 666$$

(b)   To within x percent of the true value π (see Fig. 13.5)

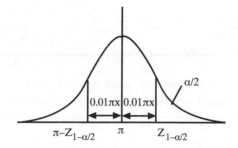

Fig. 13.5   Sampling distribution of sample proportion showing objective of the study.

The sample size (n) can in this case be calculated using the formula

$$n = \frac{z_{1-\alpha/2}^2(1-\pi)}{\pi(0.01x)^2} \tag{13.12}$$

Again using $\pi = 0.5$ produces a conservative n value.

Example 13.6

Suppose that we now wish to estimate π to within 5% of π again with 99% confidence.

Solution

$$n = \frac{(2.58)^2(1-0.5)}{(0.5)(0.01 \times 5)^2} \approx 2663$$

13.3.5   Sample size for estimating the difference between two proportions ($\pi_1 - \pi_2$)

(a)   To within x percentage points of π the true value ($\pi_1 - \pi_2$) or π_D and using equal sample sizes in the two groups

The value n, the sample size for each group, can be calculated using the formula

$$n = \frac{z_{1-\alpha/2}^2\left[\pi_1(1-\pi_1) + \pi_2(1-\pi_2)\right]}{(0.01x)^2} \tag{13.13}$$

Example 13.7

Suppose that we wish to estimate the difference in the proportion of children with dental caries in two groups of children of different socio-economic backgrounds. If we wish to estimate that difference to within five percentage points of the true difference with 99% confidence.

Solution

$$n = \frac{2.58^2 \left[0.5(1-0.5) + 0.5(1-0.5)\right]}{(0.01 \times 5)^2} \approx 1332$$

(b)   To within x percentage points of the true value $(\pi_1 - \pi_2)$ and using sample sizes which are such than n_2 is the sample size corresponding to group 2 is kn_1 where k is a constant and n_1 corresponds to group 1

The formula to use is

$$n = \frac{z_{1-\alpha/2}^2 \left[k\pi_1(1-\pi_1) + \pi_2(1-\pi_2)\right]}{k(0.01x)^2} \qquad (13.14)$$

Example 13.8

Suppose that we are likely to be able to recruit only about 60% of the number of children in group 2 compared to group 1 in the same time period and we wish to estimate the difference in the proportion of children with dental caries as before again to within 5 percentage points of the true difference with 99% confidence.

Solution

$$n_1 = \frac{2.58^2 \left[0.5 \times 0.6(1-0.5) + 0.5(1-0.5)\right]}{0.6(0.01 \times 5)^2} \approx 1776$$

$$n_2 = 0.6n_1 = 0.6 \times 1776 \approx 1066$$

13.3.6 *Sample sizes for hypothesis testing*

When carrying out calculations to obtain sample sizes necessary for hypothesis testing the following information is required:

(1)   The significance level (α) of the test.
(2)   The minimum difference which one aims to detect.
(3)   The power required for detecting predefined difference (i.e. define β).
(4)   An estimate of the standard deviation of the response being measured or estimates of the proportions being considered.

A single population proportion

Suppose that we wish to test the hypothesis

$$H_0 : \pi = \pi_0$$
$$H_1 : \pi \neq \pi_0$$

in such a way that the risk of falsely rejecting H_0 is α and of falsely accepting H_0 when it is false and $\pi = \pi_\alpha$ is β (see Fig. 13.6).

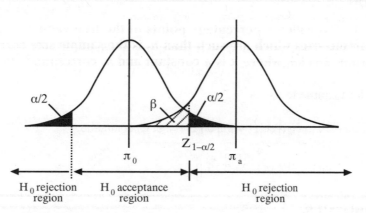

Fig. 13.6   Sampling distribution for a one sample two-sided test.

The sample size (n) required is calculated using

$$n = \frac{\left\{ z_{1-\alpha/2} \sqrt{\left[\pi_0 \left(1 - \pi_0 \right) \right]} + z_{1-\beta} \sqrt{\left[\pi_a \left(1 - \pi_a \right) \right]} \right\}^2}{\left(\pi_a - \pi_0 \right)^2} \tag{13.15}$$

Example 13.9

Suppose that we wish to test the hypothesis that the proportion of children with dental caries is 0.7 using a random sample with an α risk of 0.05 and a β risk is 0.1 if the true proportion were 0.8.

Solution

$$H_0 : \pi = 0.7$$
$$H_1 : \pi \neq 0.7$$

$$n = \frac{\left\{ 1.96 \sqrt{\left[0.7(1 - 0.7) \right]} + 1.28 \sqrt{\left[0.8(1 - 0.8) \right]} \right\}^2}{(0.8 - 0.7)^2} \approx 199$$

Difference between two population proportions

> ## Example 13.10
>
> It is estimated that 10% of young women suffer from eating disorders. In planning a study to investigate whether such disorders are more common in insulin-dependent diabetics, a group of investigators wish to determine the sample size required. Their specifications are: (1) an α level of 0.05 and (2) a 90% chance of detecting an increase of 15 percentage points in the risk of suffering from the eating disorders in the diabetic patients (Fairburn *et al.*, 1991).
>
> ## Solution
>
> The sample size required is calculated using equation
>
> $$n = \left\{ \frac{1.96\sqrt{[2(0.175)(1-0.175)]} + 1.282\sqrt{[0.1(0.9)+(0.25)(0.75)]}}{(0.1-0.25)} \right\}^2$$
>
> $= 133$ patients.
>
> Using equation to correct for violation of assumptions made:
>
> $$n' = \left(\frac{133}{4}\right)\left\{1 + \sqrt{[1+4/(133 \times 0.15)]}\right\}^2$$
>
> $= 146$

13.4 Formulae for confidence intervals

Remember that the general formula for a confidence interval (Chapter 10) is given by

$$[\text{Statistic of interest}] \pm \left[\begin{array}{l}\text{Critical value for the} \\ \text{sampling distribution}\end{array}\right]\left[\begin{array}{l}\text{Standard error of the} \\ \text{statistic of interest}\end{array}\right]$$

Therefore, for a difference between two means $(\bar{x}_1 - \bar{x}_2)$, the $100(1 - \alpha)\%$ confidence interval is given by the general formula

$$[\bar{x}_1 - \bar{x}_2] \pm [\text{Critical value}] \times \text{SE}[\bar{x}_1 - \bar{x}_2]$$

where the critical value and the standard error can be calculated from the formula in Table 13.4.

Table 13.4 Formulae for calculating sample sizes for various study designs or hypotheses.

Case	Critical value	Standard error
I		
σ_1^2 and σ_2^2 known	$z_{\alpha/2}$	$\sqrt{\sigma_1^2/n_1 + \sigma_2^2/n_2}$
Sample sizes n_1 and n_2	$z_{\alpha/2} = 1.96$ at $\alpha = 0.05$	σ_1^2 and σ_2^2 are the known population variances
Populations normally distributed or $n_1, n_2 \geq 30$		
II		
σ_1^2 and/or σ_2^2 unknown	$z_{\alpha/2}$	$\sqrt{s_1^2/n_1 + s_2^2/n_2}$
Populations normally distributed and n_1 and $n_2 \geq 30$ *or* Populations not normally distributed but n_1 and $n_2 \geq 50$		s_1^2 and s_2^2 are the sample variances
III		
σ_1^2 and/or σ_2^2 unknown but equal	$t_{\alpha/2}$ with $(n_1 + n_2 - 2)$ degrees of freedom	$\sqrt{s_p^2/n_1 + s_p^2/n_2}$
Population normally distributed n_1 and/or $n_2 < 30$		where s_p^2 = pooled estimate of variance and given by $$s_p^2 = \sqrt{\frac{(n_1-1)s_1^2 + (n_2-1)s_2^2}{(n_1+n_2-2)}}$$
IV		
σ_1^2 and/or σ_2^2 unknown and unequal	t' where $t' = t_{\alpha/2}$ with ν degrees of freedom and rounded to nearest integer	$\sqrt{s_1^2/n_1 + s_2^2/n_2}$
Populations normally distributed	$$\nu = \frac{\left(s_1^2/n_1 + s_2^2/n_2\right)^2}{\left[\dfrac{\left(s_1^2/n_1\right)^2}{n_1-1} + \dfrac{\left(s_2^2/n_2\right)^2}{n_2-1}\right]}$$	

Table 13.4   *Continued*

Case	Critical value	Standard error
V Non-normal populations but symmetric; poion variances unknown but *equal*	$t_{\alpha/2}$ with $(m_1 + m_2 - 2)$ degrees of freedom where m_1 and m_2 are the trimmed sample sizes	$\sqrt{\dfrac{(n_1-1)s_{1w}^2 + (n_2-1)s_{2w}^2}{m_1+m_2-2}}$ where s_{1w}^2 and s_{2w}^2 are the variances of the Winsorised samples
VI Non-normal populations but symmetric; population variances unknown but *unequal*	$t_{\alpha/2}$ with ν degrees of freedom where $\nu =$ $\dfrac{\left(s_{\bar{x}_{1t}}^2 + s_{\bar{x}_{2t}}^2\right)^2}{\left[\dfrac{\left(s_{\bar{x}_{1t}}^2\right)^2}{m_1-1} + \dfrac{\left(s_{\bar{x}_{2t}}^2\right)^2}{m_2-2}\right]}$ and $s_{\bar{x}_{1t}}^2 = \dfrac{s_{1w}^2}{m_1} \cdot \dfrac{(n_1-1)}{(m_1-1)}$ and $s_{\bar{x}_{2t}}^2 = \dfrac{s_{2w}^2}{m_2} \cdot \dfrac{(n_2-1)}{(m_2-1)}$	$\sqrt{s_{\bar{x}_{1t}}^2 + s_{\bar{x}_{2t}}^2}$
VII σ_1^2 and/or σ_2^2 unknown Non-symmetric populations n_1 and $n_2 < 60$		Mann-Whitney confidence interval (not covered in this book; see Neave and Worthington (1988) p. 354). The confidence interval is given by MINITAB

Chapter 14
Research Synthesis: Systematic Overviews and Metaanalysis

14.1 Objective

One of the major activities of the pharmacist is the evaluation of clinical research and its translation into clinical advice for both patients and health workers. In the past the main method for doing this was through qualitative or narrative reviews. There is now substantial empirical evidence to show that such reviews are often biased and their conclusions often misleading. To minimise bias, a systematic approach is required when reviewing the literature. Reviews undertaken with such an approach are now generally referred to as *systematic reviews*. In such reviews it is often appropriate to statistically pool the results of the relevant studies to provide improved estimates of effect. Such statistical pooling of results from published reports is termed *metaanalysis*.

Metaanalysis, then, is a component of a systematic review, although not all systematic reviews include a metaanalysis since there may not be sufficient consistent data in the research area reviewed for statistical pooling. The scheme shown below in Section 14.2 illustrates where metaanalysis fits in a systematic review.

In this chapter, the focus will be on how to pool the quantitative data. Readers interested in the broader aspects of systematic reviews are referred to two articles by the author (Li Wan Po, 1996 and 1997).

14.2 Essential steps in undertaking a systematic overview

The essential steps in a systematic overview may be summarised as follows.

Step 1
Define the primary and subobjectives of the overview.

Step 2
Define the relevant outcome measures (i.e. what is to be measured to determine efficacy or success or failure).

Step 3
Conduct a systematic retrieval of all the relevant studies.

Step 4
Perform qualitative and quantitative abstracting of the appropriate information.

Step 5
Summarise the evidence qualitatively and quantitatively by metaanalysis.

Step 6
Interpret the results to tease out important conclusions.

14.3   Statistical methods

Only a few of the basic methods of metaanalysis will be discussed from among the multitude now available.

14.3.1   *Method 1 – Dichotomous outcomes*

This method involves pooling of odds and risk ratios and risk or rate differences (see Chapter 11 for a review of these terms).

In many studies, the outcome of interest is dichotomous (e.g. death, having a myocardial infarction or not, being cured or not). Contexts in which data of this type may arise include clinical trials of drugs which are thought to prevent myocardial infarction and epidemiological studies investigating whether smoking is associated with an increase in the rate of lung cancer.

Example 14.1

To illustrate the calculations, consider the data shown in Table 14.1 which gives the results of randomised placebo-controlled clinical trials evaluating whether nicotine replacement therapy is effective in smoking cessation.

The individual studies

Each study can be written as a 2×2 contingency table (see Chapter 11) as shown in Table 14.2.

From the data given by Abelin *et al.* (1989a and 1989b) (row 1, Table 14.2) we can form the contingency table given in Table 14.3. From this table we can calculate the following statistics at the 1-year assessment point.

Odds ratio (OR)

$$= \frac{a/c}{b/d}$$

$$= 11/88 \div 17/83 \ = 0.61 \tag{14.1}$$

Risk or rate ratio (RR)

$$= \frac{a/(a+c)}{b/(b+d)}$$

$$= 11/99 \div 17/100 = 0.65 \tag{14.2}$$

Risk or rate difference (RD)

$$= b/(c+d) - a/(a+c)$$

$$= 17/100 - 11/99 = 0.059 \tag{14.3}$$

Table 14.1 Effect of nicotine patches in smoking cessation assessed by sustained abstinence at 12 months.

Reference	Nicotine replacement therapy group		Placebo control group	
	n_1	N_1	n_2	N_2
Abelin 1989a,b	17	100	11	99
Hurt 1990	9	35	8	35
Ehrsam 1991	7	56	2	56
Tonnesen 1991, 1992	25	145	6	144
ICRF 1993, 1994	76	842	53	844
Russell 1993	37	400	10	200
Sacks 1993	28	113	10	107
Kornitzer 1995	19	150	10	75
Stapleton 1995	77	800	19	400
Campbell 1996	24	115	17	119
Paoletti 1996	17	60	5	60

n_1 = number still not smoking at the end of 12 months in the nicotine replacement group; N_1 = number randomised to nicotine replacement group;
n_2 = number giving up smoking at the end of 12 months in the placebo control group; N_2 = number randomised to the placebo group.

Table 14.2 Contingency table for representing the results of a given trial.

	Treatment	
	Nicotine	Placebo
Given up smoking	a	b
Still smoking	c	d
Total	$a + c$	$b + d$

Table 14.3 Contingency table for the data given by Abelin *et al.* (1989a and 1989b) given in row 1 of Table 14.1.

	Treatment	
	Nicotine	Placebo
Given up smoking	17	11
Still smoking	83	88
Total	100	99

Number needed to treat (NNT) = 1/RD

$$= 17 \tag{14.4}$$

These results can be interpreted as the odds of retaining non-smoking status when on a placebo relative to when on a nicotine patch is 0.61. Likewise, the rate ratio (RR) gives the probability of maintaining non-smoking status when on a placebo relative to when on the nicotine patch. This is 0.65 in Abelin *et al.*'s study. The rate difference (RD) gives the difference in proportion of individuals maintaining non-smoking status between placebo and the nicotine patch. Abelin *et al.*'s data suggest an RD 0.059 in favour of the patch. This can be translated into the number needed to treat (NNT) by taking its inverse. In this example, the NNT is 17 which can be interpreted as on average, 17 subjects have to use nicotine patches for one more subject to maintain non-smoking status at 1 year.

Defining the confidence interval for estimate of effect in a given study

To calculate the confidence interval round each point estimate, we need their sampling distributions. For OR and RR these are asymmetric about the mean and to normalise the data we resort to taking the log transformation.

So, to find the confidence interval for the odds ratio of a given study, for OR, the standard error (SE) of the natural logarithm ($\log_e$) of OR, is given by

$$SE[\log_e(OR)] = \sqrt{\left(\frac{1}{a} + \frac{1}{b} + \frac{1}{c} + \frac{1}{d}\right)}$$

$$= \sqrt{\left(\frac{1}{17} + \frac{1}{11} + \frac{1}{83} + \frac{1}{88}\right)}$$

$$= 0.42 \tag{14.5}$$

The 95% confidence interval is given by

$$\log_e(OR) \pm 1.96 \times SE[\log_e(OR)] \tag{14.6}$$

In terms of the OR itself the 95% confidence interval is given by

$$e^{\log_e(OR) - 1.96 \times SE[\log_e(or)]}, \qquad e^{\log_e(OR) + 1.96 \times SE[\log_e(OR)]} \tag{14.7}$$

or

(0.27, 1.38)

Pooling of odds ratios – fixed effects

We assign a weight (w_1) to each estimate of effect [$\log_e(OR_i)$, in this case] and calculate the pooled estimate of effect Y_p as follows:

$$Y_p = \sum w_i y_i / \sum w_i \tag{14.8}$$

where $i = 1, 2, \ldots, k$

For the 11 studies shown in Table 14.1 we obtain the estimates shown in Table 14.4 for the individual effects and their corresponding variance (v_i) and weights (w_i). Also shown are the random effects weights, w_i^* (see Equation 14.17).

Table 14.4   Estimated $\log_e$ odds ratios and associated variance and weights for the 11 studies shown in Table 14.1.

Study	$\log_e$(OR)	Variance[$\log_e$(OR)]	Weight (w_i)	w_i^*
Abelin 1988a,b	−0.49381	0.173144	5.7755	4.2848
Hurt 1990	−0.15552	0.311610	3.2091	2.6893
Ehrsam 1991	−1.34993	0.681784	1.4667	1.34
Tonnesen 1991, 1992	−1.56688	0.222246	4.4995	3.5400
ICRF 1993, 1994	−0.39256	0.034596	28.9055	10.5450
Russell 1993	−0.66095	0.135045	7.4049	5.1208
Sacks 1993	−1.16168	0.157788	6.3376	4.5866
Kornitzer 1995	0.05896	0.175650	5.6931	4.2393
Stapleton 1995	−0.75876	0.069626	14.3624	7.7004
Campbell 1996	−0.45895	0.121283	8.2452	5.5091
Paoletti 1996	−1.46991	0.300261	3.3304	2.7739

The variance of Y_p is given by

$$Y_p = 1 \Big/ \sum w_i \tag{14.9}$$

and the associated 95% confidence interval by

$$Y_p \pm 1.96 \times \sqrt{V_p} \tag{14.10}$$

In our Example 14.1 the confidence interval for $\log_e$(OR) is given by

$$95\%\text{CI for } \log_e(OR_p) = -0.618922 \pm 1.96 \times 0.105863$$

$$\text{or } -0.82641, \ -0.41143$$

In terms of odds ratio, the 95% confidence interval is given by

$$95\%\text{CI for OR} = \left[e^{-0.82641}, \ e^{-0.41143} \right]$$

or

$$[0.43762, 0.662702)$$

and a print estimate of 0.53853.

Pooling of odds ratios – random effects

The fixed effects analysis described above assumes homogeneity with respect to effect seen in the k studies (11 in Table 14.2). To test for this, we can calculate a homogeneity statistic Q given by

$$Q = \sum w_i (y_i - y_p)^2 \tag{14.11}$$

where $i = 1, 2, \ldots, k$ and

which is distributed approximately chi square with $(k - 1)$ degrees of freedom.

Using the data in Table 14.3 and the values given in Equation 14.12, gives a Q-value of 14.49 which is not statistically significant suggesting little evidence of interstudy variation in the $\log_e(\text{OR})$ values.

However, suppose that we did find evidence of heterogeneity and wish to take this into account, we can then use a random effects model. Indeed, some authors suggest that the chi-square heterogeneity test is of low power and a random effects model is generally more appropriate so as to account for the possibility that some studies, yet to be published, have different results. Under this model, the studies being pooled are assumed to be a random sample from a larger population of studies with a mean population effect size, μ, around which each study's effect varies.

Under this model (according to DerSimonian and Laird, 1986), the interstudy variance can be calculated as

$$V_1 = (Q - (k - 1))/U \qquad \text{if} \qquad Q > k - 1 \text{ and 0 otherwise} \tag{14.12}$$

where

$$U = (k - 1)\left[\overline{w} - (S_w^2/k\overline{w})\right] \tag{14.13}$$

$$S_w^2 = \frac{1}{k-1}\left(\sum w_i^2 - k\overline{w}^2\right) \tag{14.14}$$

$$\overline{w} = \sum w_i/k \tag{14.15}$$

The random effects point (y_p) and interval estimates are then given by

$$y_p^* = \sum w_i^* y_i \bigg/ \sum w_i^* \tag{14.16}$$

$$95\%\text{CI} = y_p^* \pm 1.96 \bigg/ \sqrt{\left(\sum w_i^*\right)} \tag{14.17}$$

where

$$w_i^* = 1/(V_i + V_1) \tag{14.18}$$

In Example 14.1, Table 14.1, the pooled point and interval estimates for $\log_e(\text{OR})$ are given by

Mean pooled $\log_e(\text{OR}) = -0.66781$

95% CI for $\log_e(\text{OR})$ $= -0.93873, \; -0.39688$

95% CI for OR $= e^{-0.93873}, \; e^{-0.39688}$

$= 0.39, \; 0.67$

Confidence interval for rate ratio of a given study

Similarly for the rate ratio, the $SE[\log_e(\text{RR})]$ is given by

$$SE\left[\log_e(\text{RR})\right] = \sqrt{(q_1/N_1 P_1 + q_2/N_2 p_2)} \tag{14.19}$$

where

$$p_1 = a/(a+c) \qquad p_2 = b/(b+d) \tag{14.20}$$

and

$$q_1 = 1 - p_1 \qquad q_2 = 1 - q, \tag{14.21}$$

The 95% confidence interval of $\log_e(RR)$ is given by

$$\log_e(RR) \pm 1.96 \times SE\left[\log_e(RR)\right] \tag{14.22}$$

and in terms of RR itself, the 95% confidence interval is given by

$$e^{\log_e(RR)-1.96 \times SE[\log_e(RR)]}, \quad e^{\log_e(RR)+1.96 \times SE[\log_e(RR)]} \tag{14.23}$$

For Abelin *et al.*'s data we have the 95% confidence interval as

$$e^{0.65 - 1.96 \times 0.36}, \quad e^{0.65 + 1.96 \times 0.36}$$

or   (0.95, 3.89)

The 95% confidence interval and other statistics can be calculated for each of the 11 studies and the data are shown in Table 14.4 for the $\log_e(OR)$.

Confidence interval for rate difference of a given study

For the rate difference, the variance of the estimate for the *i*th trial is given by

$$V_i = P_{1i}(1 - P_{1i})/n_{1i} + P_{2i}/n_{2i} \tag{14.24}$$

In our example of Abelin *et al.*'s data

$$RD_i = -0.05889$$

The variance associated with this estimate is given by

$$V_i = (0.17)(0.83)/100 - (0.11111)(0.88889)/99 = 0.00241$$

The 95% confidence interval for the estimated mean rate difference RD_i is given by

95% CI for $RD_i = RD_i \pm 1.96 \times SE(RD_i)$

$$RD_i \pm 1.96 \times \sqrt{0.00241} \text{ or } [-0.155, 0.037] \tag{14.25}$$

For the first study in Table 14.1 then, the conclusion is that there is no significant difference in the proportion of subjects maintaining non-smoking status between the placebo and nicotine patch group.

The confidence interval for the estimated rate difference can similarly be found.

Pooling of risk or rate ratios – fixed effects

Using the same formulae as for the odds ratio (Equations 14.8, 14.9 and 14.10), the pooled mean estimate of the risk ratios can be calculated. Using Example 14.1 and Table 14.1 data, the following estimates are obtained

Pooled estimate of mean $\log_e(RR) = -0.54163$

95% CI for mean $\log_e(RR)$ $= -0.72778,\ -0.35548$

95% CI for mean RR $= 0.48,\ 0.70$

Pooling of risk or rate ratios – random effects

Using Equations 14.11–14.16 gives the following estimates

Pooled estimate of mean $\log_e(RR) = -0.57650$

95% CI for mean $\log_e(RR)$ $= -0.81326,\ -0.33973$

95% CI for mean RR $= 0.56,\ 0.71$

14.3.2   Method 2 – Continuous outcomes

Pooling of standardised difference between two means

Suppose that we have the results of k studies comparing the responses of two independent samples of subjects to two treatments (e.g. hypertensive agents) on a continuous response variable (e.g. blood pressure). We can express the result in terms of the pooled standard deviation (S_p) of the responses to the two treatments as shown below for the ith study.

$$Y_y = \left(\overline{X}_{1i} - \overline{X}_{2i}\right)/S_p \tag{14.26}$$

The variance, V_i, of Y_i is approximately equal to

$$V_i = \left(n_{1i} + n_{2i}\right)/n_{1i}n_{2i} \tag{14.27}$$

For each of the k studies we can calculate the corresponding effect size, Y_i, and the associated variance, V_i.

To obtain a pooled effect size, we can use the inverse variance as the weight for each study as before.

$$w_i = 1/V_i \tag{14.28}$$

Using Equations 14.8, 14.9 and 14.10, the point estimate for the standardised effect size and the associated confidence interval can be calculated as before.

Appendices

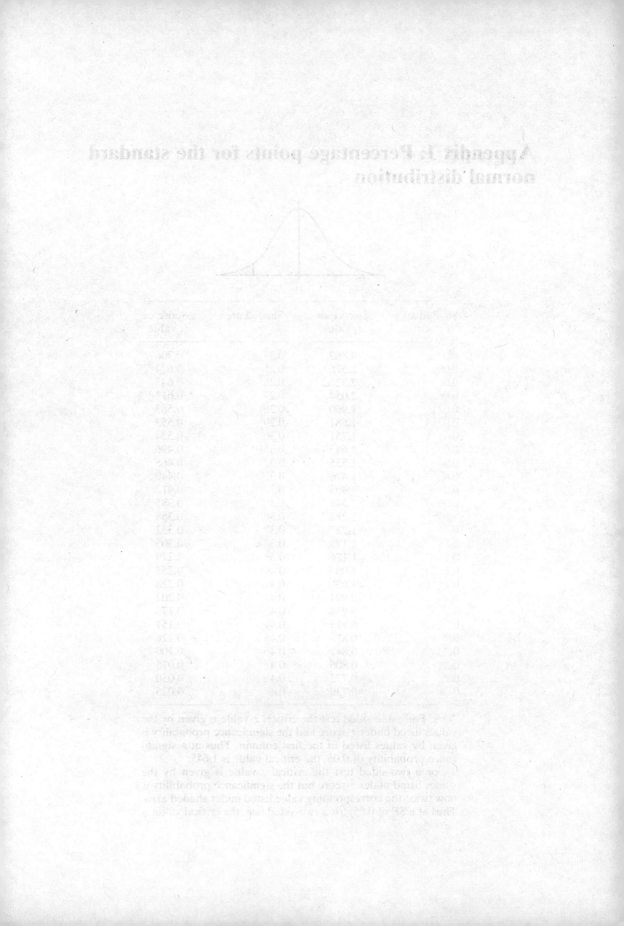

Appendix 1: Percentage points for the standard normal distribution

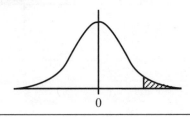

Shaded area	z-score or z_1 value	Shaded area	z-score or z_1 value
0.00	4.862	0.24	0.706
0.005	2.576	0.25	0.674
0.01	2.326	0.26	0.643
0.02	2.054	0.27	0.613
0.025	1.960	0.28	0.583
0.03	1.881	0.29	0.553
0.04	1.751	0.30	0.524
0.05	1.645	0.31	0.496
0.06	1.555	0.32	0.468
0.07	1.476	0.33	0.440
0.08	1.405	0.34	0.412
0.09	1.341	0.35	0.385
0.10	1.282	0.36	0.358
0.11	1.227	0.37	0.332
0.12	1.175	0.38	0.305
0.13	1.126	0.39	0.279
0.14	1.080	0.40	0.253
0.15	1.036	0.41	0.228
0.16	0.994	0.42	0.202
0.17	0.954	0.43	0.176
0.18	0.915	0.44	0.151
0.19	0.878	0.45	0.126
0.20	0.841	0.46	0.100
0.21	0.806	0.47	0.075
0.22	0.772	0.48	0.050
0.23	0.739	0.49	0.025

Note: For a one-sided test the critical z-value is given by the values listed under z-score and the significance probability is given by values listed in the first column. Thus at a significance probability of 0.05, the critical value is 1.645.

For a two-sided test the critical z-value is given by the values listed under z-score but the significance probability is now twice the corresponding value listed under shaded area. Thus at a SP of 0.05, for a two-sided test, the critical value is 1.960.

Appendix 2: Percentage points for the *t*-distribution

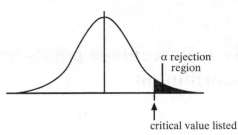

α rejection region

critical value listed

Degrees of freedom, ν	Area to the right				Degrees of freedom, ν	Area to the right			
	0.05	0.025	0.01	0.005		0.05	0.025	0.01	0.005
1	6.314	12.706	31.821	63.657	52	1.675	2.007	2.400	2.674
2	2.920	4.303	6.965	9.925	53	1.674	2.006	2.399	2.672
3	2.353	3.182	4.541	5.841	54	1.674	2.005	2.397	2.670
4	2.132	2.776	3.747	4.604	55	1.673	2.004	2.396	2.668
5	2.015	2.571	3.365	4.032	56	1.673	2.003	2.395	2.667
6	1.943	2.447	3.143	3.707	57	1.672	2.003	2.394	2.665
7	1.895	2.365	2.998	3.499	58	1.672	2.002	2.392	2.663
8	1.860	2.306	2.896	3.355	59	1.671	2.001	2.391	2.662
9	1.833	2.262	2.821	3.250	60	1.671	2.000	2.390	2.660
10	1.812	2.228	2.764	3.169	61	1.670	2.000	2.389	2.659
11	1.796	2.201	2.718	3.106	62	1.670	1.999	2.388	2.658
12	1.782	2.179	2.681	3.055	63	1.669	1.998	2.387	2.656
13	1.771	2.160	2.650	3.012	64	1.669	1.998	2.386	2.655
14	1.761	2.145	2.624	2.977	65	1.669	1.997	2.385	2.654
15	1.753	2.131	2.602	2.947	66	1.668	1.997	2.384	2.652
16	1.746	2.120	2.583	2.921	67	1.668	1.996	2.383	2.651
17	1.740	2.110	2.567	2.898	68	1.668	1.996	2.382	2.650
18	1.734	2.101	2.552	2.878	69	1.667	1.995	2.382	2.649
19	1.729	2.093	2.539	2.861	70	1.667	1.994	2.381	2.648
20	1.725	2.086	1.528	2.845	71	1.667	1.994	2.380	2.647
21	1.721	2.080	2.518	2.831	72	1.666	1.994	2.379	2.646
22	1.717	2.074	2.508	2.819	73	1.666	1.993	2.379	2.645
23	1.714	2.069	2.500	2.807	74	1.666	1.993	2.378	2.644
24	1.711	2.064	2.492	2.797	75	1.665	1.992	2.377	2.643
25	1.708	2.060	2.485	2.787	76	1.665	1.992	2.376	2.642
26	1.706	2.056	2.479	2.779	77	1.665	1.991	2.376	2.641
27	1.703	2.052	2.473	2.771	78	1.665	1.991	2.375	2.640
28	1.701	2.048	2.467	2.763	79	1.664	1.991	2.375	2.640
29	1.699	2.045	2.462	2.756	80	1.664	1.990	2.374	2.639
30	1.697	2.042	2.457	2.750	81	1.664	1.990	2.373	2.638
31	1.696	2.040	2.453	2.744	82	1.664	1.989	2.373	2.637
32	1.694	2.037	2.449	2.739	83	1.663	1.989	2.372	2.636
33	1.692	2.035	2.445	2.733	84	1.663	1.989	2.372	2.636
34	1.691	2.032	2.441	2.728	85	1.663	1.988	2.371	2.635
35	1.690	2.030	2.438	2.724	86	1.663	1.988	2.371	2.634
36	1.688	2.028	2.435	2.720	87	1.663	1.988	2.370	2.634
37	1.687	2.026	2.431	2.715	88	1.663	1.987	2.370	2.633
38	1.686	2.024	2.429	2.712	89	1.662	1.987	2.369	2.632
39	1.685	2.023	2.426	2.708	90	1.662	1.987	2.369	2.632
40	1.684	2.021	2.423	2.705	91	1.662	1.986	2.368	2.631
41	1.683	2.020	2.421	2.701	92	1.662	1.986	2.368	2.630
42	1.682	2.018	2.419	2.698	93	1.661	1.986	2.367	2.630
43	1.681	2.017	2.416	2.695	94	1.661	1.986	2.367	2.629
44	1.680	2.015	2.414	2.692	95	1.661	1.985	2.366	2.629
45	1.679	2.014	2.412	2.690	96	1.661	1.985	2.366	2.628
46	1.679	2.013	2.410	2.687	97	1.661	1.985	2.365	2.628
47	1.678	2.012	2.408	2.685	98	1.661	1.985	2.365	2.627
48	1.677	2.011	2.407	2.682	99	1.660	1.984	2.365	2.626
49	1.677	2.010	2.405	2.680	100	1.660	1.984	2.364	2.626
50	1.676	2.009	2.403	2.678	128	1.657	1.979	2.356	3.155
51	1.675	2.008	2.402	2.676					

For a one-sided test at a significance probability of α the critical value is the corresponding value given in the table. For example, with 6 degrees of freedom, for a one-sided test at a significance probability of 0.05, the critical *t* value is 1.943. If, on the other hand, the test is two-sided, the critical value is 2.447.

Appendix 3: 5% percentage points for the *F*-distribution

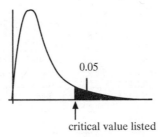

0.05

critical value listed

v_1 v_2	1	2	3	4	5	6	7	8	9	10	15	20	40
2	18.51	19.00	19.16	19.25	19.30	19.33	19.35	19.37	19.38	19.40	19.43	19.45	19.47
3	10.13	9.55	9.28	9.12	9.01	8.94	8.89	8.85	8.81	8.79	8.70	8.66	8.59
4	7.71	6.94	6.59	6.39	6.26	6.16	6.09	6.04	6.00	5.96	5.86	5.80	5.72
5	6.61	5.79	5.41	5.19	5.05	4.95	4.88	4.82	4.77	4.74	4.62	4.56	4.46
6	5.99	5.14	4.76	4.53	4.39	4.28	4.21	4.15	4.10	4.06	3.94	3.87	3.77
7	5.59	4.74	4.35	4.12	3.97	3.87	3.79	3.73	3.68	3.64	3.51	3.44	3.34
8	5.32	4.46	4.07	3.84	3.69	3.58	3.50	3.44	3.39	3.35	3.22	3.15	3.04
9	5.12	4.26	3.86	3.63	3.48	3.37	3.29	3.23	3.18	3.14	3.01	2.94	2.83
10	4.96	4.10	3.71	3.48	3.33	3.22	3.14	3.07	3.02	2.98	2.85	2.77	2.66
11	4.84	3.98	3.59	3.36	3.20	3.09	3.01	2.95	2.90	2.85	2.72	2.65	2.53
12	4.75	3.89	3.49	3.26	3.11	3.00	2.91	2.85	2.80	2.75	2.62	2.54	2.43
13	4.67	3.81	3.41	3.18	3.03	2.92	2.83	2.77	2.71	2.67	2.53	2.46	2.34
14	4.60	3.74	3.34	3.11	2.96	2.85	2.76	2.70	2.65	2.60	2.46	2.39	2.27
15	4.54	3.68	3.29	3.06	2.90	2.79	2.71	2.64	2.59	2.54	2.40	2.33	2.20
16	4.49	3.63	3.24	3.01	2.85	2.74	2.66	2.59	2.54	2.49	2.35	2.28	2.15
17	4.45	3.59	3.20	2.96	2.81	2.70	2.61	2.55	2.49	2.45	2.31	2.23	2.10
18	4.41	3.55	3.16	2.93	2.77	2.66	2.58	2.51	2.46	2.41	2.27	2.19	2.06
19	4.38	3.52	3.13	2.90	2.74	2.63	2.54	2.48	2.42	2.38	2.23	2.16	2.03
20	4.35	3.49	3.10	2.87	2.71	2.60	2.51	2.45	2.39	2.35	2.20	2.12	1.99
21	4.32	3.47	3.07	2.84	2.68	2.57	2.49	2.42	2.37	2.32	2.18	2.10	1.96
22	4.30	3.44	3.05	2.82	2.66	2.55	2.46	2.40	2.34	2.30	2.15	2.07	1.94
23	4.28	3.42	3.03	2.80	2.64	2.53	2.44	2.37	2.32	2.27	2.13	2.05	1.91
24	4.26	3.40	3.01	2.78	2.62	2.51	2.42	2.36	2.30	2.25	2.11	2.03	1.89
25	4.24	3.39	2.99	2.76	2.60	2.49	2.40	2.34	2.28	2.24	2.09	2.01	1.87
26	4.23	3.37	2.98	2.74	2.59	2.47	2.39	2.32	2.27	2.22	2.07	1.99	1.85
27	4.21	3.35	2.96	2.73	2.57	2.46	2.37	2.31	2.25	2.20	2.06	1.97	1.84
28	4.20	3.34	2.95	2.71	2.56	2.45	2.36	2.29	2.24	2.19	2.04	1.96	1.82
29	4.18	3.33	2.93	2.70	2.55	2.43	2.35	2.28	2.22	2.18	2.03	1.94	1.81
30	4.17	3.32	2.92	2.69	2.53	2.42	2.33	2.27	2.21	2.16	2.01	1.93	1.79
40	4.08	3.23	2.84	2.61	2.45	2.34	2.25	2.18	2.12	2.08	1.92	1.84	1.69

The critical values at the 5% significance level are listed in the table. For example, at this significance level the *F*-distribution with $3(v_1)$ and $40(v_2)$ degrees of freedom has a critical value of 2.84 (see Table – last entry of column 3). This is shown in the figure at the top. The shaded area gives the significance level (α) which is 0.05 in this case. More extensive tables are available in Neave (1979), or *Documenta Geigy* and many other sources.

Appendix 4: Upper percentage points for the Studentised range, $q_\alpha = (\bar{Y}_{max} - \bar{Y}_{min})/S_{\bar{Y}}$

Error df	α	p = number of								
		2	3	4	5	6	7	8	9	10
1	0.05	18.0	27.0	32.8	37.1	40.4	43.1	45.4	47.4	49.1
	0.01	90.0	135	164	186	202	216	227	237	246
2	0.05	6.09	8.3	9.8	10.9	11.7	12.4	13.0	13.5	14.0
	0.01	14.0	19.0	22.3	24.7	26.6	28.2	29.5	30.7	31.7
3	0.05	4.50	5.91	6.82	7.50	8.04	8.48	8.85	9.18	9.46
	0.01	8.26	10.6	12.2	13.3	14.2	15.0	15.6	16.2	16.7
4	0.05	3.93	5.04	5.76	6.29	6.71	7.05	7.35	7.60	7.83
	0.01	6.51	8.12	9.17	9.96	10.6	11.1	11.5	11.9	12.3
5	0.05	3.64	4.60	5.22	5.67	6.03	6.33	6.58	6.80	6.99
	0.01	5.70	6.97	7.80	8.42	8.91	9.32	9.67	9.97	10.24
6	0.05	3.46	4.43	4.90	5.31	5.63	5.89	6.12	6.32	6.49
	0.01	5.24	6.33	7.03	7.56	7.97	8.32	8.61	8.87	9.10
7	0.05	3.34	4.16	4.68	5.06	5.36	5.61	5.82	6.00	6.16
	0.01	4.95	5.92	6.54	7.01	7.37	7.68	7.94	8.17	8.37
8	0.05	3.26	4.04	4.53	4.89	5.17	5.40	5.60	5.77	5.92
	0.01	4.74	5.63	6.20	6.63	6.96	7.24	7.47	7.68	7.37
9	0.05	3.20	3.95	4.42	4.76	5.02	5.24	5.43	5.60	5.74
	0.01	4.60	5.43	5.96	6.35	6.66	6.91	7.13	7.32	7.49
10	0.05	3.15	3.88	4.33	4.65	4.91	5.12	5.30	5.46	5.60
	0.01	4.48	5.27	5.77	6.14	6.43	6.67	6.87	7.05	7.21
11	0.05	3.11	3.82	4.26	4.57	4.82	5.03	5.20	5.35	5.49
	0.01	4.39	5.14	5.62	5.97	6.25	6.48	6.67	6.84	6.99
12	0.05	3.08	3.77	4.20	4.51	4.75	4.95	5.12	5.27	5.40
	0.01	4.32	5.04	5.50	5.84	6.10	6.32	6.51	6.67	6.81
13	0.05	3.06	3.73	4.15	4.45	4.69	4.88	5.05	5.19	5.32
	0.01	4.26	4.96	5.40	5.73	5.98	6.19	6.37	6.53	6.67
14	0.05	3.03	3.70	4.11	4.41	4.64	4.83	4.99	5.13	5.25
	0.01	4.21	4.89	5.32	5.63	5.88	6.08	6.26	6.41	6.54
15	0.05	3.01	3.67	4.08	4.37	4.60	4.78	4.94	5.08	5.20
	0.01	4.17	4.83	5.25	5.56	5.80	5.99	6.16	6.31	6.44
16	0.05	3.00	3.65	4.05	4.33	4.56	4.74	4.90	5.03	5.15
	0.01	4.13	4.78	5.19	5.49	5.72	5.92	6.08	6.22	6.35
17	0.05	2.98	3.63	4.02	4.30	4.52	4.71	4.86	4.99	5.11
	0.01	4.10	4.74	5.14	5.43	5.66	5.85	6.01	6.15	6.27
18	0.05	2.97	3.61	4.00	4.28	4.49	4.67	4.82	4.96	5.07
	0.01	4.07	4.70	5.09	5.38	5.60	5.79	5.94	6.08	6.20
19	0.05	2.96	3.59	3.98	4.25	4.47	4.65	4.79	4.92	5.04
	0.01	4.05	4.67	5.05	5.33	5.55	5.73	5.89	6.02	6.14
20	0.05	2.95	3.58	3.96	4.32	4.45	4.62	4.77	4.90	5.01
	0.01	4.02	4.64	5.02	5.29	5.51	5.69	5.84	5.97	6.09
24	0.05	2.92	3.53	3.90	4.17	4.37	4.54	4.68	4.81	4.92
	0.01	3.96	4.54	4.91	5.17	5.37	5.54	5.69	5.81	5.92
30	0.05	2.89	3.49	3.84	4.10	4.30	4.46	4.60	4.72	4.83
	0.01	3.89	4.45	4.80	5.05	5.24	5.40	5.54	5.65	5.76
40	0.05	2.86	3.44	3.79	4.04	4.23	4.39	4.52	4.63	4.74
	0.01	3.82	4.37	4.70	4.93	5.11	5.27	5.39	5.50	5.60
60	0.05	2.83	3.40	3.74	3.98	4.16	4.31	4.44	4.55	4.65
	0.01	3.76	4.28	4.60	4.82	4.99	5.13	5.25	5.36	5.45
120	0.05	2.80	3.36	3.69	3.92	4.10	4.24	4.36	4.48	4.56
	0.01	3.70	4.20	4.50	4.71	4.87	5.01	5.12	5.21	5.30
∞	0.05	2.77	3.31	3.63	3.86	4.03	4.17	4.29	4.39	4.47
	0.01	3.64	4.12	4.40	4.60	4.76	4.88	4.99	5.08	5.16

Appendix 5: Percentage points for the chi-square distribution

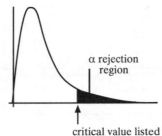

α rejection region

critical value listed

Degrees of freedom, ν	Shaded area			
	0.975	0.050	0.025	0.010
1	0.000	3.842	5.024	6.635
2	0.0501	5.992	7.378	9.210
3	0.216	7.815	9.348	11.345
4	0.484	9.488	11.143	13.277
5	0.831	11.071	12.833	15.086
6	1.237	12.592	14.449	16.812
7	1.690	14.067	16.013	18.475
8	2.180	15.507	17.535	20.090
9	2.700	16.919	19.023	21.666
10	3.247	18.307	20.483	23.209
11	3.816	19.675	21.920	24.725
12	4.404	21.026	23.337	26.217
13	5.009	22.362	24.736	27.688
14	5.629	23.685	26.119	29.141
15	6.262	24.996	27.488	30.578
16	6.908	26.296	28.845	32.000
17	7.564	27.587	30.191	33.409
18	8.231	28.869	31.526	34.805
19	8.907	30.144	32.852	36.191
20	9.591	31.410	34.170	37.566
21	10.283	32.671	35.479	38.932
22	10.982	33.924	36.781	40.289
23	11.689	35.173	38.076	41.638
24	12.401	36.415	39.364	42.980
25	13.120	37.653	40.647	44.314
26	13.844	38.885	41.923	45.642
27	14.573	40.113	43.195	46.963
28	15.308	41.337	44.461	48.278
29	16.047	42.557	45.722	49.588
30	16.791	43.773	46.979	50.892

Appendix 6: Critical values for the Spearman's rank correlation coefficient

Number of pairs of ranks	Critical value of rank correlation r_s coefficient in a one-tail test	
	Significance level	
	0.05	0.01
6	0.829	0.943
7	0.714	0.893
8	0.643	0.833
9	0.600	0.783
10	0.564	0.746

For samples of pairs bigger than 10 in size calculate the test statistic

$$t = r_s \sqrt{\left(\frac{n-2}{1-r_s^2} \right)}$$

where r is the coefficient and n is the sample size and test against the critical one-tail t value with $(n-2)$ degrees of freedom.

Appendix 7: Critical values at the 5% significance level for the Mann-Whitney test

One-sided test

Larger sample size	Smaller sample size																			
	1	2	3	4	5	6	7	8	9	10	11	12	13	14	15	16	17	18	19	20
1	–	–																		
2	–	–																		
3	–	–	0																	
4	–	–	0	1																
5	–	0	1	2	4															
6	–	0	2	3	5	7														
7	–	0	2	4	6	8	11													
8	–	1	3	5	8	10	13	15												
9	–	1	3	6	9	12	15	18	21											
10	–	1	4	7	11	14	17	20	24	27										
11	–	1	5	8	12	16	19	23	27	31	34									
12	–	2	5	9	13	17	21	26	30	34	38	42								
13	–	2	6	10	15	19	24	28	33	37	42	47	51							
14	–	2	7	11	16	21	26	31	36	41	46	51	56	61						
15	–	3	7	12	18	23	28	33	39	44	50	55	61	66	72					
16	–	3	8	14	19	25	30	36	42	48	54	60	65	71	77	83				
17	–	3	9	15	20	26	33	39	45	51	57	64	70	77	83	89	96			
18	–	4	9	16	22	28	35	41	48	55	61	68	75	82	88	95	102	109		
19	–	4	10	17	23	30	37	44	51	58	65	72	80	87	94	101	109	116	123	
20	–	4	11	18	25	32	39	47	54	62	69	77	84	92	100	107	115	123	130	138

Two-sided test

Larger sample size	Smaller sample size																			
	1	2	3	4	5	6	7	8	9	10	11	12	13	14	15	16	17	18	19	20
1	–																			
2	–	–																		
3	–	–	–																	
4	–	–	–	0																
5	–	–	0	1	2															
6	–	–	1	2	3	5														
7	–	–	1	3	5	6	8													
8	–	0	2	4	6	8	10	13												
9	–	0	2	4	7	10	12	15	17											
10	–	0	3	5	8	11	14	17	20	23										
11	–	0	3	6	9	13	16	19	23	26	30									
12	–	1	4	7	11	14	18	22	26	29	33	37								
13	–	1	4	8	12	16	20	24	28	33	37	41	45							
14	–	1	5	9	13	17	22	26	31	36	40	45	50	55						
15	–	1	5	10	14	19	24	29	34	39	44	49	54	59	64					
16	–	1	6	11	15	21	26	31	37	42	47	53	59	64	70	75				
17	–	2	6	11	17	22	28	34	39	45	51	57	63	69	75	81	87			
18	–	2	7	12	18	24	30	36	42	48	55	61	67	74	80	86	93	99		
19	–	2	7	13	19	25	32	38	45	52	58	65	72	78	85	92	99	106	113	
20	–	2	8	14	20	27	34	41	48	55	62	69	76	83	90	98	105	112	119	127

The critical regions include all values smaller than those listed in the tables.

Appendix 8: Critical values for the Wilcoxon matched-pairs signed-ranks test

Number of pairs of data values which were ranked	Maximum value smaller sum of ranks can have and still be significant in a one-tail test	
	Level of significance	
	0.05	0.01
6	2	sample too small
7	3	0
8	5	1
9	8	3
10	10	4
11	13	7
12	17	9
13	21	12
14	25	15
15	30	19
16	36	24

If the number of pairs which were ranked is greater than 16 the z score

$$z = \frac{m(m+1)/4 - T - 0.5}{\sqrt{[m(m+1)(2m+1)/24]}}$$

where m is the number of ranks and T is the smaller sum of ranks, can be used in a one-tail test.

Appendix 9: Critical values for the sign test

The tabulated values are for the two-sided test. For a one-sided test simply divide the α value by two to obtain the corresponding significance level.

For large sample sizes the critical value can be approximated by

$$n = \frac{1}{2}\left(n - z_{1-\alpha/2}\sqrt{n-1}\right)$$

α / n	10%	5%	2%	1%	α / n	10%	5%	2%	1%	α / n	10%	5%	2%	1%	α / n	10%	5%	2%	1%
1	–	–	–	–	26	8	7	6	6	51	19	18	16	15	76	30	28	27	26
2	–	–	–	–	27	8	7	7	6	52	19	18	17	16	77	30	29	27	26
3	–	–	–	–	28	9	8	7	6	53	20	18	17	16	78	31	29	28	27
4	–	–	–	–	29	9	8	7	7	54	20	19	18	17	79	31	30	28	27
5	0	–	–	–	30	10	9	8	7	55	20	19	18	17	80	32	30	29	28
6	0	0	–	–	31	10	9	8	7	56	21	20	18	17	81	32	31	29	28
7	0	0	0	–	32	10	9	8	8	57	21	20	19	18	82	33	31	30	28
8	1	0	0	0	33	11	10	9	8	58	22	21	19	18	83	33	32	30	29
9	1	1	0	0	34	11	10	9	9	59	22	21	20	19	84	33	32	30	29
10	1	1	0	0	35	12	11	10	9	60	23	21	20	19	85	34	32	31	30
11	2	1	1	0	36	12	11	10	9	61	23	22	20	20	86	34	33	31	30
12	2	2	1	1	37	13	12	10	10	62	24	22	21	20	87	35	33	32	31
13	3	2	1	1	38	13	12	11	10	63	24	23	21	20	88	35	34	32	31
14	3	2	2	1	39	13	12	11	11	64	24	23	22	21	89	36	34	33	31
15	3	3	2	2	40	14	13	12	11	65	25	24	22	21	90	36	35	33	32
16	4	3	2	2	41	14	13	12	11	66	25	24	23	22	91	37	35	33	32
17	4	4	3	2	42	15	14	13	12	67	26	25	23	22	92	37	36	34	33
18	5	4	3	3	43	15	14	13	12	68	26	25	23	22	93	38	36	34	33
19	5	4	4	3	44	16	15	13	13	69	27	25	24	23	94	38	37	35	34
20	5	5	4	3	45	16	15	14	13	70	27	26	24	23	95	38	37	35	34
21	6	5	4	4	46	16	15	14	13	71	28	26	25	24	96	39	37	36	34
22	6	5	5	4	47	17	16	15	14	72	28	27	25	24	97	39	38	36	35
23	7	6	5	4	48	17	16	15	14	73	28	27	26	25	98	40	38	37	35
24	7	6	5	5	49	18	17	15	15	74	29	28	26	25	99	40	39	37	36
25	7	7	6	5	50	18	17	16	15	75	29	28	26	25	100	41	39	37	36

Appendix 10: Table of random numbers from the standard normal distribution

2.38773	−0.07817	−0.48617	−0.88440	−1.52888	−0.57063	−1.13067
0.90767	0.06787	0.24414	1.16845	0.76268	−0.00779	−0.97337
0.29470	−0.51140	0.34696	−1.99818	−0.14937	1.67093	−0.46942
0.82568	−1.81009	−0.75322	−1.27142	−1.10709	−2.00931	0.47386
−1.07159	−2.09678	0.29608	−1.16933	−1.75511	−1.38302	−0.55172
1.41597	−0.52536	−0.28553	−0.36034	0.43792	−1.32256	1.46248
−0.74051	−0.58515	−0.08915	1.63359	−0.36480	1.87378	0.06244
1.61289	−0.71053	0.04101	0.34498	−0.76271	0.42913	−0.75321
−0.00459	−0.57318	0.36418	−0.17964	−0.76342	−2.54342	−0.16495
1.73528	0.47074	−1.27153	−1.78722	2.84584	1.88102	0.97421
0.88426	0.39415	0.65508	1.31432	−0.84344	0.35072	−0.40126
−0.75688	0.04357	−0.55375	0.66459	−0.55597	−1.65658	0.34004
−0.58171	−1.08170	1.66132	−0.16689	−2.17561	0.95528	0.54492
−1.24895	−0.02264	−0.83657	−0.37270	0.19824	1.71586	−1.82447
−0.33020	2.16277	−1.21706	−0.29219	0.85666	1.37152	0.57216
0.24430	1.42474	−0.39104	0.66339	−0.24151	0.08841	−0.33382
0.34714	−0.30248	0.00269	−0.02227	−3.17846	−0.01201	−0.05955
−1.13797	−1.63156	−1.45656	−1.41197	−1.20248	−0.51625	1.08632
1.03033	−0.52599	−1.05528	−0.41683	0.34131	−0.29853	−0.28436
1.14365	−0.49738	−1.12499	−2.02416	0.56510	−1.86865	0.33843
−1.37223	−0.46051	1.14534	−0.94356	0.21882	−1.20619	−0.53593
−1.21197	0.91685	−1.31581	0.31929	1.73081	0.40929	−0.32509
−0.77393	−0.61729	1.96009	−0.97097	0.15359	−1.31479	−0.44274
−1.70587	0.24047	0.58718	−0.64669	−0.68700	0.07061	0.15695
−0.59402	0.22499	0.06414	−1.42117	−0.99693	−1.22232	−0.00920
−1.15023	2.35542	−0.74361	−0.47123	1.38919	−0.48005	0.17913
−1.41562	−1.90663	−0.67833	0.77113	0.23686	1.40005	1.14826
0.92824	−0.93276	−0.98135	1.11828	0.23904	−0.01643	−2.05391
1.73495	0.18685	0.64233	−1.33077	0.97407	−0.09450	0.92007
0.84278	0.10887	0.53979	−0.98730	1.03815	1.52913	−1.51841
1.81454	−0.37333	0.63417	0.53375	−0.54073	−1.37404	1.50658
0.15686	−1.02031	−0.35355	−1.31299	−0.47471	−0.25099	1.39451
0.48624	−0.70198	1.99945	0.01950	1.73842	0.33359	0.82684
0.22887	−1.38205	−1.43149	1.16574	0.60043	−0.01227	−1.53352
0.26892	−0.35919	0.77024	0.11894	0.67492	1.00039	0.02423
3.02827	1.33471	−0.22900	0.60490	−0.53628	0.30793	0.62674
−0.94379	0.45324	−0.76623	−1.67079	−1.11382	1.86364	−0.44976
−0.56124	1.93578	0.90598	0.60643	0.00713	−0.77126	−0.53426
0.67126	0.10185	0.56431	−1.21956	−0.18018	−0.66850	−0.55431
0.34361	−0.93030	−0.17647	−0.26880	0.31802	−1.75160	−0.03996
0.49179	0.42988	−0.05321	0.79286	0.35205	−0.52249	2.33159
1.45277	0.08954	1.89280	0.51163	0.17021	0.55135	0.43711
0.34613	−0.08288	−0.04225	0.20437	−0.48002	−0.11751	0.03803
0.82658	−0.60226	−0.02591	0.39407	−0.74038	−0.68737	−0.70390
−1.36873	−1.61858	0.39925	0.01424	0.18226	−0.56515	−0.54429

Appendix 11: Table of random integers

7	8	2	6	8	9	2	6	2	3	6	1	5	3	5
3	5	2	9	1	1	8	5	4	1	4	6	7	3	4
9	7	5	7	8	0	0	8	0	4	7	8	5	8	9
8	1	6	0	9	5	2	2	1	5	9	8	9	5	9
0	6	7	7	4	9	5	0	6	1	7	8	0	1	6
4	8	9	7	9	5	4	8	7	3	6	1	9	8	3
4	8	1	6	0	8	6	1	5	0	6	0	8	3	9
4	7	1	5	1	7	6	1	1	1	5	9	8	9	7
7	6	7	6	7	1	2	1	6	8	6	3	3	4	6
9	4	8	3	2	1	0	4	5	7	4	9	5	6	0
1	2	6	9	5	4	5	1	3	5	8	4	8	7	5
6	0	4	8	9	3	1	3	7	8	5	5	6	5	5
8	4	4	3	2	9	7	5	9	0	9	5	1	7	4
1	1	5	7	7	8	7	5	9	5	4	0	0	7	1
5	8	8	3	9	8	1	7	2	0	6	7	3	5	6
5	6	9	9	1	6	7	3	4	6	8	9	7	6	4
4	9	8	2	4	2	3	4	3	9	3	6	3	0	3
5	2	9	1	8	3	4	2	2	8	6	1	3	5	8
1	0	0	0	4	4	5	0	9	6	1	7	6	8	6
4	1	7	3	0	8	9	3	3	5	9	8	4	1	3
7	0	2	4	6	1	6	7	5	4	4	8	0	8	2
1	3	1	3	8	9	7	8	4	9	0	6	7	0	4
4	2	3	2	5	9	5	4	2	2	7	2	2	8	1
6	2	3	9	2	5	5	7	4	8	3	5	7	7	9
0	8	5	0	8	1	0	0	4	5	7	5	8	9	6
7	8	8	3	8	7	9	2	5	3	0	3	9	8	7
2	8	3	2	8	4	6	1	9	3	5	9	4	7	5
4	6	6	2	0	3	9	9	8	4	5	3	0	5	0
9	0	6	2	8	8	4	1	5	9	4	1	9	9	3
4	2	9	5	7	3	2	9	9	0	4	4	2	6	0
7	8	3	7	1	1	5	3	3	2	0	3	7	1	1
8	7	4	4	1	5	5	7	5	0	4	4	6	5	3
6	6	3	7	0	9	6	0	4	8	6	1	6	9	1

Appendix 12: Table of critical values for Kendall's rank correlation coefficient

n	σ_2			
	10%	5%	2%	1%
1	–	–	–	–
2	–	–	–	–
3	–	–	–	–
4	1.000	–	–	–
5	0.800	1.000	1.000	–
6	0.733	0.876	0.867	1.000
7	0.619	0.714	0.810	0.905
8	0.571	0.643	0.714	0.786
9	0.500	0.556	0.667	0.722
10	0.467	0.511	0.600	0.644
11	0.418	0.491	0.564	0.600
12	0.394	0.455	0.546	0.576
13	0.359	0.436	0.513	0.564
14	0.363	0.407	0.473	0.517
15	0.333	0.391	0.467	0.505
16	0.317	0.383	0.433	0.483
17	0.309	0.368	0.427	0.471
18	0.294	0.346	0.412	0.451
19	0.287	0.333	0.392	0.439
20	0.274	0.326	0.379	0.421
21	0.267	0.314	0.371	0.410
22	0.264	0.307	0.359	0.394
23	0.257	0.296	0.352	0.391
24	0.246	0.290	0.341	0.377
25	0.240	0.287	0.333	0.367
26	0.237	0.280	0.329	0.360
27	0.231	0.271	0.322	0.356
28	0.228	0.265	0.312	0.344
29	0.222	0.261	0.310	0.340
30	0.218	0.255	0.301	0.333
31	0.213	0.252	0.295	0.325
32	0.210	0.246	0.290	0.323
33	0.205	0.242	0.288	0.314
34	0.201	0.237	0.280	0.312
35	0.197	0.234	0.277	0.304
36	0.194	0.232	0.273	0.302
37	0.192	0.228	0.267	0.297
38	0.189	0.223	0.263	0.292
39	0.188	0.220	0.261	0.287
40	0.185	0.218	0.256	0.285
41	0.181	0.215	0.254	0.281
42	0.178	0.213	0.250	0.275
43	0.176	0.209	0.247	0.274
44	0.173	0.207	0.243	0.269
45	0.172	0.204	0.240	0.267
46	0.169	0.202	0.239	0.264
47	0.167	0.199	0.236	0.260
48	0.167	0.197	0.232	0.257
49	0.163	0.196	0.230	0.253
50	0.162	0.192	0.228	0.251

Appendix 13: Calculating probabilities for observed test statistics using series approximations

The following formulae may be used for calculating probabilities associated with observed test statistics from various commonly used probability distributions.

Probabilities for test statistics

The normal distribution N(0, 1)

The area to the right of a Z score under the standard normal curve is

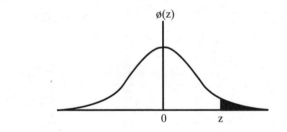

$$P(Z \text{ score} \geq z) = \int_{z}^{\infty} \frac{e^{-z^2/2}}{\sqrt{(2\pi)}} \, dz$$

$$= 0.5 - \frac{1}{\sqrt{(2\pi)}} \left(z - \frac{z^3}{3.2} + \frac{z^5}{5.2^2.2!} - \frac{z^7}{7.2^3.3!} + \dots \right)$$

$Z \sim N(0, 1^2)$

The chi-squared distribution χ_v^2

The area under its distribution curve to the right of a chi-squared value x with v degrees of freedom is

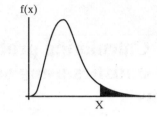

$$P\left(\chi^2 \geq x\right) = \frac{\int_x^\infty x^{(v-2)/2} e^{-x/2} dx}{\int_0^\infty x^{(v-2)/2} e^{-x/2} dx}$$

$$= 2 \left(\text{area to right of } \sqrt{x} \text{ on standard normal curve}\right)$$

$$+ \frac{e^{-x/2}}{\sqrt{\pi}} \left(\frac{(x/2)^{1/2}}{\dfrac{1}{2} \cdot} + \frac{(x/2)^{3/2}}{\dfrac{3}{2} \cdot \dfrac{1}{2}} + \frac{(x/2)^{5/2}}{\dfrac{5}{2} \cdot \dfrac{3}{2} \cdot \dfrac{1}{2}} + \cdots \right.$$

$$\left. + \frac{(x/2)^{(v/2)-1}}{(v/2-1)(v./2-2) \cdots \dfrac{1}{2}} \right) \text{ if v is odd.}$$

$$= e^{-x/2} \left(1 + \frac{(x/2)^1}{1!} + \frac{(x/2)^2}{2!} + \cdots + \frac{(x/2)^{(v/2)-1}}{(v/2-1)!} \right) \text{ if v is even.}$$

The *F*-distribution F_{v_1,v_2}

The area under its distribution curve to the right of the ration F of a variance with v_1 degrees of freedom divided by a variance with v_2 degrees of freedom is

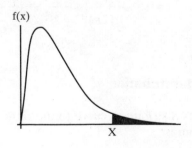

$$P(F \geq x) = \frac{\int_{0}^{w} w^{(v_2/2)-1}(1-w)^{(v_1/2)-1}\,dw}{\int_{0}^{1} w^{(v_2/2)-1}(1-w)^{(v_1/2)-1}\,dw}$$

where $w = v_2/(v_2 + v_1 x)$

The integrals can be expressed as a series of powers of w:

$$\frac{w^{(v_2/2)-1}}{v_1/2}\left(1-(1-w)^{v_1/2}\right) - \frac{[(v_2/2)-1]w^{v_2/2}}{v_2/2} + \frac{[(v_2/2)-1][(v_1/2)-1]w^{(v_2/2)+1}}{[(v_2/2)+1]2!}$$

$$- \frac{[(v_2/2)-1][(v_1/2)-1][(v_1/2)-2]w^{v_2/2}}{[(v_2/2)+2]3!} + \cdots$$

t-distribution with v degrees of freedom (t_v)

t-values from the t distribution with v degrees of freedom are related to F-values from the F-distribution with 1 and v degrees of freedom as follows:

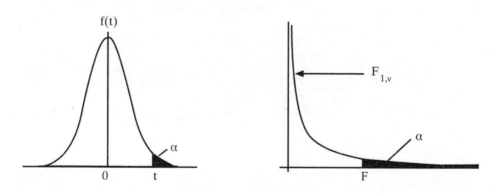

$$t_v^2 = F_{1,v}$$

$P(T \geq t)$ = shaded area
$\equiv P(F \geq t^2)$ with $F_{1,v}$ degrees of freedom.

Therefore the same formula used to approximate F probabilities may be used to calculate t probabilities. Simply put $v_1 = 1$ and $v_2 = v$ into the formula and take the square root of the answer.

Appendix 14: Some transformations to normalise skewed data

Each dot represents 22 points

```
 .
 :
 :
 ::
 ::
 ::
 :::
 :::::
 :::::
 ::::::::
 ::::::::::::::::::::::::           .      .      .       ..
+---------+---------+---------+---------+---------+---
```

Log transformation

Each dot represents 4 points

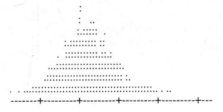

Invert (-) and then
log transformation

Each dot represents 22 points

```
                                                  .
                                                  :
                                                  ::
                                                  ::
                                                  :::
                                                  :::::
                                                  ::::::
                             .    .      .    .::::::::::::::::
         +---------+---------+---------+---------+---------+
```

Each dot represents 5 points

Square root
transformation √x

Each dot represents 2 points

Invert (-) and square
root (√x) transformation

Each dot represents 5 points

References and Further Reading

Abelin, T., Buehler, A., Muller, P. and Vesanen, K. (1989a) Controlled trial of transdermal nicotine patch tobacco withdrawal. *Lancet*, **i**, 7–10.

Abelin, T., Ehrsam, R., Buhler-Teichert, A., Imhof, P.R., Muller, P., Thommen, A. and Vesanen, K. (1989b) Effectiveness of a transdermal nicotine system in smoking cessation studies. *Methods and Findings in Experimental and Clinical Pharmacology*, **11**, 205–14.

Agresti, A. (1990) *Categorical Data Analysis*. John Wiley & Sons: New York.

Al-sereiti, M.R., Coakes, R.L., O'Sullivan, D.P.D. and Turner, P. (1989) A comparison of the ocular hypotensive effect of 0.025% bromocriptine and 0.25% timolol eye-drops in normal human volunteers. *British Journal of Clinical Pharmacology*, **28**, 443–7.

Altman, D.G. (1991) *Practical Statistics for Medical Research*. Chapman and Hall: London.

Armitage, P. and Berry, G. (1987) *Statistical Methods in Medical Research*, 2nd edn. Blackwell Scientific Publications: Oxford.

Bates, D.M. (1988) *Non-linear Regression Analysis and its Applications*. John Wiley & Sons: New York.

Bland, M. (1987) *Introduction to Medical Statistics*. Oxford University Press: Oxford.

Bowlt, C. and Tiplady, P. (1989) Radioiodine in human thyroid glands and incidence of thyroid cancer in Cumbria. *British Medical Journal*, **299**, 301–2.

Box, G.E.P. and Tiao, G.C. (1973) *Bayesian Inference in Statistical Analysis*. Addison-Wesley: Reading.

Box, G.E.P., Hunter, W.G. and Hunter, J.S. (1978) *Statistics for Experimenters*. John Wiley & Sons: New York.

Bradford-Hill, A. (1965) The environment and disease: association or causation. *Journal of the Royal Society of Medicine*, **58**, 295–300.

Campbell, I.A., Prescott, R.J., Tjeder-Burton, S.M. (1996) Transdermal nicotine plus support in patients attending hospital with smoking-related diseases: a placebo-controlled study. *Respiratory Medicine*, **90**, 47–51.

Cohen, J. (1960) A coefficient of agreement for nominal scales. *Educational and Psychological Measurement*, **20**, 37–46.

Cohen, J. (1968) Weighted Kappa. *Psychological Bulletin*, **70**, 213–20.

Crowder, M.J. and Hand, D.J. (1990) *Analysis of Repeated Measures*. Chapman and Hall: London.

Dale, G., Fleetwood, J.A., Weddell, A. *et al.* (1987) β endorphin: a factor in fun run collapse? *British Medical Journal*, **297**, 1004.

DerSimonian, R. and Laird, N. (1986) Metaanalysis in clinical trials. *Controlled Clinical Trials*, **7**, 177–88.

Ehrsam, R.E., Buhler, A., Muller, P., Mauli, D., Schumacher, P.M., Howald, H. and Imhof, P.R. (1991) Transdermal nicotine as an aid towards abstinence in young smokers. *Schweizerische Rundschau fur Medizin/Praxis*, **80**, 145–50.

Fairburn, C.G., Peveler, R.C., Davies, B., Mann, J.I. and Mayon, R.D. (1991) Eating disorders in young adults with insulin-dependent diabetes mellitus. *British Medical Journal*, **303**, 17–20.

Fleiss, J.L. (1971) Measuring nominal scale agreement among many raters. *Psychological Bulletin*, **76**, 378–82.

Goodman, L.A. and Kruskal, W.H. (1954) Measures of association for cross-classifications. *Journal of the American Statistical Association*, **49**, 732–64.

Goodman, L.A. and Kruskal, W.H. (1972) Measures of association for cross classifications – simplification of asymptotic variances. *Journal of the American Statistical Association*, **67**, 415–21.

Hedges, A., Hills, M., Maclay, W.P., Newman-Taylor, A.J. and Turner, P. (1971) Some central and peripheral effects of meclastine, a new antihistamine drug, in man. *Journal of Clinical Pharmacology*, **2**, 112–19.

Hurt, R.D., Lauger, G.G., Offord, K.P., Kottke, T.E. and Dale, L.C. (1990) Nicotine-replacement therapy with use of a transdermal nicotine patch – a randomized double-blind placebo-controlled trial. *Mayo Clinic Proceedings*, **65**, 1529–37.

Iman, R. and Conover, W.J. (1979) The use of the rank transform in regression. *Technometrics*, **21**, 499–509.

ICRF (Imperial Cancer Research Fund General Practice Research Group) (1993) Effectiveness of a nicotine patch in helping people stop smoking: results of a randomised trial in general practice. *British Medical Journal*, **306**, 1304–8.

ICRF (Imperial Cancer Research Fund General Practice Research Group) (1994) Randomized trial of nicotine patches in general practice: results at one year. *British Medical Journal*, **308**, 1476–7.

Kendall, M.G. (1970) *Rank Correlation Methods*. Griffin: London.

Kingdom, J.C.P., Kelly, T., Maclean, A.B. and McAllister, E.J. (1991) Rapid one-step urine test for human chorionic gonadotrophin in evaluating suspected complicatiens of early pregnancy. *British Medical Journal*, **302**, 1308–11.

Kornitzer, M., Boutsen, M., Dramaix, M., Thijs, J. and Gustavsson, G. (1995) Combined use of nicotine patch in smoking cessation: A placebo-controlled clinical trial. *Preventive Medicine*, **24**, 41–7.

Landis, J.R. and Koch G.G. (1977) The measurement of observer agreement for categorical data. *Biometrics*, **33**, 159–74.

Lemeshow, S., Hosmer Jr, D.W., Klar, J. and Lwanga, S.K. (1990) *Adequacy of Sample Size in Health Studies*. John Wiley & Sons: New York.

Li Wan Po, A. (1996) Evidence-based pharmacotherapy. *Pharmaceutical Journal*, **256**, 308–12.

Li Wan Po, A. (1997) A practical guide to undertaking a systematic overview. *Pharmaceutical Journal*, **258**, 518–20.

Neave, H.R. (1979) *Elementary Statistics Tables*. George Allen & Unwin: London.

Neave, H.R. and Worthington, P.L. (1988) *Distribution-free Tests*. Unwin Hyman: London.

Paoletti, P., Fornai, E., Maggiorelli, F., *et al.* (1996) Importance of baseline cotinine plasma values in smoking cessation: results from a double blind study with nicotine patch. *European Respiratory Journal*, **9**, 643–51.

Ratkowsky, D.A. (1989) *Handbook of Non-linear Regression Models*. Marcel Dekker Inc.: New York.

Russell, M.A.H., Stapleton, J.A., Feyerabend, C., Wiseman, S.M., Gustavsson, G., Sawe, U. and Connor, P. (1993) Targeting heavy smoking in general practice: randomised controlled trial of transdermal nicotine patches. *British Medical Journal*, **306**, 1308–12.

Sacks, D.P.L., Sawe, U. and Leischow, S.J. (1993) Effectiveness of a 16-hour transdermal nitcotine patch in a medical practice setting without intensive group counselling. *Archives of Internal Medicine*, **153**, 1881–90.

Schultz, T.W. (1987) The use of the ionisation constant (pKa) in selecting models of toxicity in phenols. *Ecotoxicology and Environmental Safety*, **14**, 178–83.

Siegel, S. and Castellan, Jr. N.J. (1988) *Nonparametric Statistics*, 2nd edn. McGraw Hill: New York.

Stapleton, J.A., Russel, M.A.H., Feyerabend, C., *et al.* (1995) Dose effects and predictors of outcome in a randomized trial of transdermal nicotine patches in general practice. *Addiction*, **90**, 31–42.

Stork, E. (1990) *Minitab Users' Group Newsletter*, **11**, 3–5.

Tabachnick, B.G., and Fidell, L.S. (1989) *Using Multivariate Statistics*, 2nd edn. Harper and Row: New York.

Tonnesen, P., Norregaard, J., Simonsen, K. and Sawe, U. (1991) A double-blind trial of a 16-hour transdermal nicotine patch in smoking cessation. *New England Journal of Medicine*, **325**, 311–15.

Tonnesen, P., Norregaard, J. and Sawe, U. (1992) Two-year outcome in a smoking cessation trial with a nicotine patch. *Journal of Smoking Related Diseases*, **3**, 241–5.

Yates, F. (1934) Contingency tables involving small numbers and the χ^2 test. *Journal of the Royal Statistical Society*, Supplement 1, 217–35.

Index

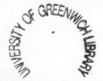